The ACL Solution

Prevention and Recovery for Sports' Most Devastating Knee Injury

Robert G. Marx, MD

with

Grethe Myklebust, PT, PhD

and

Brian W. Boyle

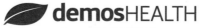 **demos**HEALTH

NEW YORK

Visit our website at www.demoshealth.com

All patient anecdotes in this book are factual. Names have been changed to protect patient privacy.

All photos appear courtesy of Nina Drapacz.

ISBN: 9781936303335
e-book ISBN: 9781617051135

Acquisitions Editor: Noreen Henson
Compositor: Diacritech

Medical information provided by Demos Health, in the absence of a visit with a health care professional, must be considered as an educational service only. This book is not designed to replace a physician's independent judgment about the appropriateness or risks of a procedure or therapy for a given patient. Our purpose is to provide you with information that will help you make your own health care decisions.

The information and opinions provided here are believed to be accurate and sound, based on the best judgment available to the authors, editors, and publisher, but readers who fail to consult appropriate health authorities assume the risk of injuries. The publisher is not responsible for errors or omissions. The editors and publisher welcome any reader to report to the publisher any discrepancies or inaccuracies noticed. *5036 3885 11/12*

Library of Congress Cataloging-in-Publication Data

CIP data is available from the Library of Congress.

Special discounts on bulk quantities of Demos Health books are available to corporations, professional associations, pharmaceutical companies, health care organizations, and other qualifying groups. For details, please contact:

Special Sales Department
Demos Medical Publishing, LLC
11 West 42nd Street, 15th Floor
New York, NY 10036
Phone: 800-532-8663 or 212-683-0072
Fax: 212-941-7842
E-mail: rsantana@demosmedpub.com

Printed in the United States of America by Bang Printing.
12 13 14 15 / 5 4 3

Contents

Foreword

The simple title of this book belies an epidemic that is taking place in schools, on basketball courts, and within families across the country. As the head women's basketball coach at Yale University for the past seven years now, I can tell you firsthand that ACL injuries wreak havoc on seasons, self-esteem, athletic careers and physical health. During the 2012–2013 season, 4 players out of thirteen on the roster will be former victims of ACL injuries—which sadly, is not an unusual ratio on a college women's basketball team. Call any basketball coach and they will tell you that the threat of the injury floats in the back of their minds during every practice and game of the season. When any of us coaches see a player crumple to the floor in the telltale response to an ACL injury, our hearts sink. For me personally, it doesn't matter if the player is on our team or the opponent's, the sadness is the same as I know the pain, frustration, and long months of recovery ahead.

For coaches, players and parents, the injury that is so prevalent also remains largely a mystery. For years I have wondered about the injury and ways to prevent it from occurring, often switching up off-season training routines or lifting regimens. Some years, we would get lucky and have a team that is ACL-injury free for an extended time. I would find myself thinking back on those seasons trying to somehow pinpoint what we did right or better than in the years we had injuries. It seemed to always be a guessing game. In this book, Dr. Marx has finally laid out, in an easy to understand and entertaining way, how these injuries occur and, most importantly, possible methods of prevention. This book is a must-read for athletic trainers and strength coaches across the country. Parents and players should also take note, as in the desire to be the best, the importance of knowing your body's functions and limits should come into play, so that beyond the college quest, there can be a healthy and mobile existence for years to come.

Women's athletics have come a long way over the last several decades and more women are getting involved in sports, not just in school, but also as a lifetime pursuit. As this number continues to increase, understanding how ACL injuries happen and how to best prevent and treat them will be critical to ensuring competitive and healthy play. The next evolution of women's athletics is going to include taking control of an injury that devastates athletes and prevents them from reaching their full potential. Dr. Marx is fulfilling an important role in this evolution, by identifying the ACL epidemic for what it is, and providing a guidebook for athletes to take back control of their own destiny. As a coach AND a mother of a female basketball player, I can tell you this education is long overdue.

Chris Gobrecht

Joel E. Smilow Head Coach of Women's Basketball

Yale University

New Haven, Connecticut

Acknowledgments

I would like to thank my wife Rena for her unwavering support, guidance and understanding over many years and whose love has been a source of inspiration to me. I am also thankful for the encouragement of my daughters Ella and Hannah, who are now somewhat expert in this field as well. Dr. Grethe Myklebust was a fantastic partner in this project and her knowledge and expertise were essential to bring forward the critical elements of injury prevention. Brian Boyle was a pleasure to work with, and if he becomes half as good of a doctor as he is a writer, he will help many people for many years. I thank Nina Drapacz for her patience and expertise as a photographer. Our close friends Jamie and Sam Lipman were fantastic models for the photographs, not only for their good looks, but their physical condition that allowed for the many re-takes needed to get the images just right. I am grateful to my good friend Richard Ellenson who encouraged me to start the writing process and whose creative genius helped me get going. I am thankful for the excellent work of my research assistant Lana Verkuil who put the book together. I am also grateful to her predecessor Kaitlyn Lillemoe who helped with the initial stages. I appreciate Dave Allen's work helping write the book proposal that got us started. I thank Lauren Hirshowitz who allowed us to use her photograph (wearing number 6 on the cover) which was taken nine months after I did her ACL reconstruction, now over ten years ago. I thank my office manager Maria Dedvukaj and my surgical coordinator Candice Miller who keep my life organized. I appreciate the work of the staff at Demos including Tom Hastings and Dana Bigelow, and particularly thank Noreen Henson for her support and flexibility. Last, but certainly not least, I am very grateful to my agent Marilyn Allen. Without her enthusiasm for the prevention of injury, this book may have never found a publisher.

Robert G. Marx, MD

New York, New York

I would like to thank Dr. Robert Marx for inviting me take part in this project. Meeting Bob at a conference in Israel some years ago was the start of this project for me. To meet an orthopedic surgeon who was so interested in the prevention of ACL injuries was fantastic. The fact that many ACL injuries can be prevented was something he wanted "everyone" to benefit from, and "knowledge translation" is what this book is really all about. I also thank all my colleagues and co-authors at the Oslo Trauma Research Center for a great and inspiring environment.

Grethe Myklebust, PT, PhD

Oslo, Norway

INTRODUCTION

Fields of Pain

THE MORGANS USED TO BE LIKE so many upper middle-class families in the United States today: their lives revolved around sports. On most evenings, Mr. and Mrs. Morgan had to make arrangements to pick up their triplets (two girls and a boy) from basketball or soccer practice, or from a game. And their weekends were spent shuttling their teenage daughters and son all over the New York metro area from tournament to tournament. But that all changed in the summer of 2007, when Michelle, one of their daughters, limped off the soccer field with an apparent left knee sprain after trying to change directions hard to avoid a defender.

After resting for a month, in which she cycled, swam and did some light jogging with little discomfort, Michelle returned to the soccer field. But so did the pain, especially as she tried to change direction on the knee. An MRI test several weeks later revealed a complete tear to the knee's anterior cruciate ligament, or ACL as it's more commonly known, and also a tear to her lateral meniscus. Michelle, all of 14 at the time, was in need of reconstructive ACL surgery.

As an orthopedic surgeon at New York City's Hospital for Special Surgery, I see girls like Michelle all the time. I perform ACL reconstructions on hundreds of knees every year. But even I was distraught at what I saw seven months later—that's when Michelle's sister, Amanda, paid a visit to my office. She had stopped suddenly on the basketball court and felt a sharp pain in her right knee. Unable to return to the game, her knee started to swell, and that's when her parents suspected that she may have incurred the same injury as her sister. An MRI a short time later revealed their worst fears: another ACL tear.

The family's misfortunes weren't over, however. After rehabbing for eight months and recovering nicely from a patellar tendon autograft ACL reconstruction in her right knee, Amanda had returned to soccer, even scoring a game-winning goal for her team in one of her first games back. Unfortunately, later in the same game, her healthy left knee suddenly twisted inward, and she felt a pop. There was no contact from another player, but the force thrust on her ACL was powerful, and she had torn it as well. The Morgan family had a total of three ACL reconstructions in less than two years.

What happened to the Morgan sisters is all too common today. There are an estimated 41 million American kids playing competitive youth sports today, and estimates run as high as 200,000 ACL surgeries per year in the U.S. alone[1,2], a large percentage of which are being performed on the knees of prepubescent kids. I have performed ACL reconstruction surgery on children as young as seven. We have an epidemic on our hands, but one you probably haven't heard about on the news. That might seem strange, given that kids have been playing sports for a long time, and the anterior cruciate ligament has certainly been around for just as long. But there is an explanation, and it lies in the recent history of youth sports.

"Back when I was a young man..." We've all heard yarns that start this way, perhaps a grandfather's claim that his voyage to school was uphill both ways and riddled with hail the size of golf balls. But we're skeptical, aren't we? And we ask ourselves, "Was it really all that different back then?"

I'm here to tell you that it was different back then, at least in the world of youth sports, but it wasn't necessarily harder. In fact, in many ways, it was easier. Forty years ago, when I was a child athlete, organized sports and weekday practices were not the norm. Travel teams were very rare. If you didn't measure up, you got picked last for the street hockey team and maybe had to sit on the curb for a while, not rejected outright to look on as your buddies boarded airplanes bound for tournaments in faraway lands. Athletic young people face an entirely different situation these days.

Like so many other spheres of our lives, youth athletics have been developed, honed, and refined over the decades. It only makes sense: if you put more time into something, you will get better at it. It has always been true for surgeons; why not for a twelve-year-old soccer player? And so that twelve-year-old is now expected to attend practice four to five times in a week, perform competitively in a match, take a day to rest (maybe), and do it again the next week.

Nor is there a significant seasonal break for many young people, as they are expected to practice their sport year-round. Perhaps I should say that they *want* to practice their sport year-round, driven by joy and passion, though any adult ought to understand the close relationship between a young person's wants and the wants of the adults around him. We could speculate on root causes—college athletic scholarships are more competitive than ever, and higher education does not come cheap. But, regardless of the motivating forces, the reality is intense.

It is also downright dangerous. There is no free lunch. The human body has limits, no matter what the age, and pushing it to those limits will have consequences that do not end when the buzzer does. These consequences can be devastating with effects that can last a lifetime. The truth is that trophies and scholarships come at the expense of the very core that allows young people to do what they do so well: *move*. Ligaments, tendons, and cartilage are being ripped apart on playing fields across the country in the name of competition. The ACL is most often the one these athletes sacrifice. Cut faster, pivot more suddenly, jump higher and land harder, we ask of our young athletes, as they ask it of themselves. And suddenly, your son or daughter is injured and can cut, pivot, and jump no more.

Indeed, the problem is particularly alarming for females. ACL tears have been increasing in number across the board, but the explosion among young women in athletics is simply staggering. Though not all of the causes are entirely understood, one of them is: females are playing more sports. Regardless of the demographic into which you fall, if you are not playing sports, you are not at significant risk for an ACL tear. As soon as you walk onto the field or court, that is no longer the case.

The 1960s were a time when young women were taking courses in home economics and typing, while their male peers whizzed baseballs at each other. This is no longer the case, and we owe that in part to Title XV of the Education Amendments of 1972, the law which amended Title IX of the Civil Rights Act of 1964. Though the original statute does not explicitly deal with athletics, this amended Title IX is most widely known for the way it has affected the role of females in high school and collegiate sports. Title IX provides for equality between the sexes in all educational activities at federally funded institutions, and athletic programs fall under that umbrella. Because the language of Title IX is sparse, its implementation over the decades has been met with resistance—most notably that spearheaded by Senator John Tower in 1974—and required several rounds of legislative clarification. As recently as 1994, the Equity in Athletics Disclosure Act went into effect, which requires institutions to make available information like male and female roster sizes, allowing better compliance monitoring. While there is hopefully none among us who laments the effectiveness of Title IX in furthering gender equality, more females in sport means more ACL tears among young women.

But young women are certainly not the only ones at risk. In fact, *young people* are not the only ones at risk. Just as young females have joined their male peers on athletic fields across the nation, adults have joined their more youthful brethren. As with young females, the change is a good one on the whole. Adults are living healthier lifestyles into their later years, staying active. Personal fitness is now a part of adult culture in a way that our parents would never have dreamed of a few decades ago. People are running, skiing and sending tennis balls across the net well into their fifties, sixties, and beyond. Not only are people staying more involved in athletics generally, but they are participating in ever more aggressive sports even as they age. That is, there aren't just more middle-aged joggers on the road; there are moms and dads on soccer and rugby fields every Sunday afternoon. The extent to which adults are putting themselves at risk for ACL tear is unprecedented.

Even worse, we're talking about a major *injury*, a random, traumatic event which would seem to be hard to predict—and it is. Some conditions have warning signs. If your cholesterol and blood pressure are high and you have a family history of heart disease, it may be a good idea to visit the cardiologist. The same is true of many other conditions in medicine. However, when it comes to the ACL, although some people may be at higher risk, we don't know precisely who they are, and it's not as though the knee produces warning signs in an individual whose athletic career could be over after the next play.

If adults and youths alike are tearing their ACLs left and right, we should figure out the best way to fix that ligament, right? Well, there is actually a much more effective way to deal with this problem: prevent it from happening. This may be difficult to understand since injuries are generally believed to be random events that are an unfortunate part of sport. I've described a trend toward ever greater intensity and injury risk in our youth and adult sports that doesn't look like it will change course—and it won't. Despite the conventional wisdom, many of these ACL tears are preventable, according to studies conducted by the Oslo Sports Trauma Research Center.[3-7] Dr. Bert Mandelbaum from Santa Monica[8-10] and Dr. Tim Hewett from Cincinnati and the Ohio State University,[11-14] among others, have also done outstanding research in the U.S. to document the effectiveness of prevention. Dr. Hewett also holds an annual ACL Workshop, which he started in 2002. During this symposium, participants learn to recognize the need for ACL injury prevention programs and describe techniques for screening athletes at risk for ACL injuries and programs for preventing these injuries. The scientific evidence that supports these prevention programs is now irrefutable!

We must apply the solution to everyone. In this case, the cure comes before the catastrophe, in the form of a comprehensive system of exercises to be performed by all athletes at risk. These exercises train athletes young and old how to control their own bodies to protect themselves from injuries, including ACL tears, ankle sprains and overuse injuries. That is, the program not only decreases the risk of ACL injury, but also the risk of many other injuries that keep athletes off the field. Like any skill in sport, these protective habits can be learned. The program which I will discuss later on does not simply improve general strength, ability, and balance; it actually ingrains in athletes the specific motor pathways which will keep them on the field and out of the hospital. There are certain ways to cut, change direction, and land from a jump which will tear the ACL, and there are other ways which will protect it. Athletes just need to be shown, and to practice, the right ways.

And the best part? The better athletes get at protecting themselves in these specific, carefully designed ways, the harder they can play while staying safe. These exercises can be used as an athlete's normal warm up routine; they build muscle strength, speed, and core stability, all of which contribute to athletic performance. I am not suggesting that we ask our young athletes to throttle back the intensity—even if I did, no one would listen. I am proposing a solution that would be the free lunch I claimed earlier didn't exist, were it not for the small price of a few extra minutes of practice with each training session. It has been scientifically proven to reduce the risk of ACL injury, and it is time to spread the good word.[15]

A natural question to ask is: why haven't people like me—medical professionals—been spreading the word already? The answer involves both Western doctors and Western patients. Physicians and surgeons in our society tend to focus on fixing things rather than keeping them from happening in the first place. Medical professionals are taught to think this way from the beginning of their training. Take medical school, for example, which focuses on what to do when something goes wrong, not on how to keep everything right. In my training, I spent countless hours learning about drugs, anatomy, and the pathophysiology of disease. Almost my entire training as a physician and surgeon was in the form of treatments for problems. This is true of almost all doctors in the United States, and possibly the world. Prevention is not something we tend to do, or do well, in general. Meanwhile, patients generally have no desire to change the way they live, preferring a pill or an incision over a diet or lifestyle change. In that sense, medical professionals, like any other kind, are providing the service their clients ask of them.

Naturally, it is difficult to determine which came first—the habits and expectations of the population with regard to their health, or the markedly cure-focused medical profession. And, ultimately, it's irrelevant. You might even think that the situation is fine as it is. After all, if the cures are there, why not just let people live the way they live? Why not just let Jim smoke? Why not let Rebecca jump out of the minivan and onto the soccer field without having to deal with prevention exercises?

We know that the heart isn't the same after a heart attack, even if the lucky patient survives and gets the bypass. Likewise, the knee isn't the same after an ACL tear, even if it is successfully reconstructed. I will discuss later on in greater detail the various ways in which this is true. Suffice it to say for now that if you can keep your own ACL rather than borrowing one from your own knee or a cadaver, you're better off. And if you don't *need* surgery on one of your major joints, well, you don't *want* it.

The simple fact is that, like many other realms of medicine and surgery, sports medicine and orthopedics cannot offer the perfect cure. Prevention is the panacea, and it's so easy to incorporate into a standard warm-up routine. Life isn't full of no-brainers—situations are not usually black-and-white—but this is one of them. Do you buckle up before putting your car into gear? Maybe the better question is this: do you buckle your *kids* up?

I hope you do, but perhaps this analogy isn't adequate. Allow me to ask a question that is more clear: would you enter a war zone without a protective flack jacket? If the answer is no, then these prevention exercises should be on your to-do list. The comparison is *not* ridiculous precisely because ACL injury rates *are* ridiculous. Ask any high school athlete what a myocardial infarction is, and he'll probably just give you a blank stare. Ask the same kid what an ACL is, and, suddenly, you're talking to a kid who sounds like an orthopedic surgeon! Why? Because one hand probably doesn't have enough fingers on it to count off the number of people he knows who have torn that ligament. It's a minefield out there—suit up.

Unfortunately, the prevention program is not to ACL injury what the vaccine was to polio. As long as competitive sports continue to exist, athletes young and old will push themselves to the limit—and then beyond it. We wouldn't have it any other way, would we?

I wrote this book for two reasons: not just to present an approach to ACL injury prevention, but to consolidate in one place what the Internet offers only in fragmented form to those who have already injured themselves. At this point, most of us are aware that the World Wide Web will tell us pretty much anything we want to know about anything. ACL injury, and what to do about it, is no exception. While the first word we might use to describe the Internet is "vast," the second would be—or at least should be—"unreliable."

They say that art may exist only for its own sake. If art is what you're after, then, I would point you to the aisle lined with books that have more pages, fewer pictures, and names on the spines that sound Russian. This book is not art. It exists not for itself, but for the generation of young athletes who may play without fear, and for those already injured, that they may recover quickly and safely. Most importantly, the exercises and information in this book can be applied to youth, high school, college, and professional athletes to decrease the rate of injury in sport. Ideally, this can be accomplished by making the prevention exercises a part of the athlete's warm up routine, or the child's gym class in school.

It will become clear as you read further that ACL injury forces patients, families, and clinicians to confront an array of decisions that may be daunting. And while there is no substitute for a doctor who knows what she's doing, medical professionals do not dictate the course of care. Patients, and the ones who love them, can do no better than to equip themselves with accurate information placed in a context that makes it *useful*. That's what this book ought to be, and I hope that you find it so.

CHAPTER ONE

Anatomy and Function of the Knee

ANATOMY IS A GREAT PLACE TO START when it comes to matters of the human body, especially those which fall under the umbrella of orthopedic surgery. If you know the parts of the knee and how they function in concert to produce the movements we take for granted every day, you can better understand the myriad ways in which the system can fail to function properly. The great thing about anatomy is that, unlike so many other aspects of medicine, things are just the way the standard text says they are. Exceptions may seem to arise more frequently, but only for brief moments. I can think of one patient whose lateral meniscus—a structure I'll discuss later in this chapter—had disappeared by a mechanism I could only imagine was magical; it just wasn't there.[16] But, sure enough, during surgery, we observed a trace of the tissue dangling in view, just enough to be pulled by a probe. What followed was a magic trick on its own: as a magician slowly pulls out of his nose a handkerchief that couldn't possibly have fit in there, we yanked on that piece of tissue until, little by little, the entire lateral meniscus revealed itself. It had flipped over and was hiding in the back of the knee. The patient, Greg Vance, was the victim of a violent basketball injury that had not only torn his ACL and sheared a large piece of cartilage off the end of his femur, but had also severely altered the anatomy of his lateral meniscus.

This brief anecdote highlights the only thing that can really fly in the face of an anatomy textbook: trauma. Your ability to find Fort Lauderdale depends only on the accuracy of the map in your glove compartment or your GPS, and your sense of direction, unless a hurricane has relocated the place a half-mile up the beach. The surgeon's ability to find the ACL, or any other structure in the knee, depends only on the accuracy of her anatomical knowledge (hopefully, the textbook is no longer necessary) and, well, sense of direction, unless trauma—or a previous surgeon—has moved it.

That's what makes revision surgery so challenging and rewarding for the experienced surgeon: the ACL graft is not always where it should be. Even when the original graft that tore was in the correct position, the surgery can still be demanding. In some cases, the original screws must be removed and perhaps replaced by screws comprised of absorbable plastic polymers and hydroxyapatite, which will form new bone, before new tunnels are drilled for the replacement graft. That primary surgery is routine in comparison to complex revision ACL surgery makes the point yet clearer: anatomy—the stuff you were born with—doesn't change. Here, I'll cover the basics of knee anatomy.

THE KNEE IS A HINGE JOINT that connects the upper leg bone (femur) to the lower leg bone (tibia). That part, you probably knew already. There are several important components to knee anatomy, including the ends of these two bones, articular cartilage, meniscus, ligaments, hamstrings, and the extensor mechanism.

The ligaments of the knee are extremely important to its function, because the shapes of the bones of the knee do not contribute significantly to its stability. Consider the knee in contrast to the hip. The hip, a ball-and-socket joint, involves a great deal of bony conformity. That is, the bones fit together like puzzle pieces, the round head of the femur held in place by the concave acetabulum of the pelvis. The knee, a hinge joint, does not have anywhere near this degree of bony conformity. While the top of the tibia has two areas (the tibial plateau), against which rest the convex bony structures at the bottom of the femur, it is the ligaments which provide the vast majority of the knee's stability. There are four major ligaments in the knee: the anterior cruciate ligament, posterior cruciate ligament, medial collateral ligament, and lateral (fibular) collateral ligament.

Unlike the other ligaments, the ACL is entirely within the knee joint. It passes from the lateral part of the end of the femur and through the center of the knee, to the front, or anterior region of the tibia. It is this anatomical position which accounts for two key characteristics of the ACL: its crucial role in pivoting and cutting and its poor healing capacity. All structures truly within the knee joint are bathed in synovial fluid, and the ACL is no exception. For this reason, blood has a harder time reaching the ACL to allow for healing. When blood cannot reach a part of the body, that part will not heal effectively.

Cutting and pivoting activities place a great deal of force on the knee, and the ACL's unique position makes it responsible for maintaining the knee's integrity against that force. It is important to note that "cutting" and "pivoting" refer to specific kinds of knee motions. We are not talking simply about high-force activities, but a specific kind of movement which results in tears of the ACL in particular. This kind of movement is common enough in sports like basketball, soccer, volleyball, racquetball, football, handball, squash, and lacrosse to make the ACL the most frequently torn ligament of them all. It is worth describing here, as an understanding of the movement which puts the ACL at risk is crucial to an understanding of the exercises which can save it.

ACL tears occur when you plant your foot on the ground and attempt to rotate your body in relation to that planted foot, placing your weight on it. This creates a twisting force across the knee joint, which the ACL must absorb. When the ACL cannot cope with that force, it ruptures. Note that the ACL will not tear when the foot is in the air; the *planting* of the foot is a crucial element of the movement which threatens the ACL. It makes sense, then, that sports which are played on high-grip surfaces, like basketball, or with shoes with cleats which help to create a high-grip relationship between the foot and the ground, like in soccer, put athletes at risk for ACL tear. Similarly, ACL tears only occur on the ski slope if the ski binding fails to release, allowing the ski to pull the foot in an awkward direction and creating the same twisting force on the knee.

We've all heard the classic injury story as told by a skier: "My ski turned out as I fell, the binding didn't release, my knee twisted, and I felt a pop. My knee swelled up and the ski patrol took me down." The attributes that make a ski so great for straight-line stability on snow also allow it to exert a huge amount of torque, or twisting force, on the knee—that is, if the binding doesn't let go first. That's why skiers typically stress their ACLs the most on skiing moguls or race courses, both of which call for tight bindings just to keep the skis on while maintaining directional control. In fact, the Norwegian group led by Dr. Roald Bahr studied the mechanism of ACL tear in professional skiers.[17] They described a "slip-catch" mechanism where the knee is bent in to a "knock-knee position," which you will hear more about later in the book. In fact this mechanism is very similar anatomically to what happens to the knee when the ACL tears from soccer and basketball injuries.

This is the kind of knowledge that can tip off a salesperson that he's dealing with a doctor when we're renting skis. Doctors don't want to tear an ACL any more than the next person; in fact, the people in my line of work see so many ACL injuries that you might even call us paranoid. I think "informed" sounds better.

I said to the salesperson preparing my rental skis: "Please make the bindings as loose as possible—just tight enough that the skis don't fall off when I turn." He gave me a knowing stare—the look you'd expect from a man who couldn't have adjusted fewer than seven-thousand bindings in his career—and posed the question, "Are you an orthopedic surgeon?"

"How did you know," I asked him, taken aback.

"Because only one person has ever made that request before, and he was an orthopedic surgeon. He told me the only times he saw someone tear their ACL skiing was when their bindings didn't release." Too loose and you'll fall over on each turn as your skis release, too tight and it could be your ACL instead.

Tight bindings or not, the mechanism of ACL injury is the same, regardless of the sport during which it takes place. Whether executing a turn on skis, landing from a jump down a staircase, or pivoting to aim for the basket, the knee is generally bent slightly and turned inward toward the other knee in what is referred to as a "valgus" position.[17-19] Rotation and shear forces across the knee, when in this position, are typically what tear the ACL.

WHILE THE ACL IS THE FOCUS of this book, it is only one part of a system of ligaments which work together to provide structure to the inherently unstable knee joint. The posterior cruciate ligament, or PCL, runs through the knee in an orientation opposite that of the ACL. That is, the ACL and PCL would appear together as a cruciform shape if viewed from the front of the knee. The PCL is a large, robust ligament that tears only when subjected to a force quite different from the one which would rupture an ACL: a direct blow to the flexed knee. A typical example is a frontal automobile impact, which can force the dashboard into the driver's and front passenger's knees as they are bent in a sitting position. This overwhelms the PCL's ability to resist rearward displacement of the tibia in relation to the femur. Unlike the ACL, the PCL is not entirely immersed in the synovium of the joint, affording it a more substantial blood supply that brings with it some healing capacity; it can be treated without surgery in some cases.

The medial collateral ligament, or MCL, is more commonly injured than the PCL. In fact, it is the ligament most commonly injured in association with the ACL—but can heal more easily on its own, as it runs between the femur and tibia on the inner, or medial, side of the knee. It has a rich blood supply because it does not lie within the knee joint itself. The MCL is more broad and band-like than cylindrical and cord-like and consists of superficial, deep, and posterior oblique components. More important than these anatomic details is the function of the MCL: it resists forces which would push the knee too far inward, toward the other knee. In other words, it is the ligament which prevents the knock-kneed stance. Skiing is one of the sports which most commonly injure the MCL, and it is easy to see why, if we consider the movements involved in carving from side-to-side down a mountain, legs almost parallel to the ground and skis digging into the snow. These forces come together to push the knee into the knock knee position, which the MCL must either flex to absorb or else ultimately rupture.

The lateral collateral ligament, also known as the fibular collateral or FCL, plays a role similar to that of the MCL but is located on the outside of the knee and therefore stabilizes the joint against forces that would create a bow-legged stance. Other lateral side structures include the popliteofibular ligament, popliteus tendon, and posterolateral capsule, all of which come together to make up the posterolateral corner, a complex network of important stabilizers that sometimes requires reconstruction in severe multi-ligament knee injuries.[20-23]

There are two menisci in the knee, one situated on the lateral side (outside) and one on the medial side (inside). Each is c-shaped and rests between the femur and tibia. Both the lateral meniscus and medial meniscus are composed of fibrocartilage, which is soft enough to absorb energy but firm enough to withstand a great deal of force without deforming or tearing. These properties make the meniscus an effective shock absorber within the knee. Think of it as a disc that provides padding to protect the cartilage on the end of both the femur and tibia. If the meniscus tears and loses its ability to function as a shock absorber, the load on the cartilage at the ends of the bones increases, and the risk of arthritis (which is loss of that cartilage) goes up dramatically. Meniscus tears are much more common in knees that have a torn ACL, making the injury even more devastating.

Cartilage on the ends of the bone within a joint is referred to as articular cartilage. It is the smooth, shiny material that we find on the end of a chicken bone. It is the breakdown or loss of articular cartilage which leads to arthritis. Arthritis indicates that there is less cartilage to absorb the force of walking, running, and just moving, imparting more pressure on the bone itself. Although cartilage has no nerves, bones are richly innervated, which is why arthritis can be so painful. Rupture of the ACL can accelerate the development of arthritis, leading to further problems years later.

Now is when it should become clear to you why we've been discussing the knee's anatomical structures in a book that focuses on the ACL. The goal is not to offer a mere anatomy lesson, but to help illustrate a relationship among the elements in the knee that makes ACL tear an even more unsettling prospect. We mentioned in the introduction that the knee is not the same after an ACL tear, and the reason involves both the menisci and the articular cartilage.

An ACL-deficient knee can "give way," or come out of alignment, particularly during cutting and pivoting movements like the ones described earlier. Remember that the ligaments are what ensure the knee's anatomical conformation; weaken or rupture one of them, and the femur and tibia are no longer sufficiently related to each other. This "giving way" can tear either of the menisci or both, which is painful and can require further surgery to remove the torn piece and alleviate the discomfort. It has been shown that a loss of meniscus can lead to arthritis.[24-26] This process is intuitive given the anatomy outlined above. The meniscus rests between the two bones which fall out of their proper anatomical position during the giving way episode, making it susceptible to tearing; and when the shock absorber is compromised, the articular cartilage is subjected to greater force and can degenerate more quickly. Degeneration of articular cartilage is arthritis and it is well established that arthritis is more common in people who have torn their ACL.[27,28]

Bones, ligaments, menisci, and cartilage, however, are not the only components of the knee. Muscles, tendons, and other soft tissues also contribute to its structure. Particularly important is the extensor mechanism, which consists of the quadriceps muscles on the front of the upper leg, the kneecap (patella), and the patellar tendon (the tissue that connects the knee cap to the lower leg). In addition to its function as a motor unit that allows us to perform daily functions like standing up, the extensor mechanism provides dynamic stability, helping to hold the knee in position during motion. Also vital are the hamstring muscles in the back of the knee.

As its name suggests, the extensor mechanism enables extension of the knee, or straightening of the leg. Its function originates in the quadriceps muscles which attach to the patella through the quadriceps tendon. A tendon is a piece of tissue that attaches muscle to bone and therefore makes the muscle effective: a muscle fires, pulls on a tendon, which pulls on a bone, and the body moves. The patella, in turn, attaches to the lower leg bone (tibia) through the patellar tendon which therefore transfers the quadriceps' pulling force to the tibia. It is this purpose of the patellar tendon which has lead to its misnomer. The patellar tendon should actually be called the patellar ligament, as ligaments connect bone to bone, while tendons, as mentioned before, connect muscle to bone. The patellar tendon is so named for its function in relation to the quadriceps, as it allows this muscle group to exact a force on the tibia, merely by pulling on the knee cap (patella).

The patella is one example of a sesamoid bone, which is a bone that sits within a tendon. Why does it exist? The answer can be found in high school physics: leverage. If a single tendon ran from the quadriceps to the tibia, the extensor mechanism would have very little leverage with the knee in a bent position. The patella increases the mechanical advantage of this system by effectively lengthening its lever arms.

To completely understand knee stability, however, we must venture even beyond the knee itself. The hamstrings—located in the back of the knee and responsible for its bending—cross both the hip and the knee joint, creating a relationship between hip stability and knee stability. In fact, the hip and the core—the muscles of the abdomen and lower back—are important to knee stability regardless of any direct anatomical connection to the knee. If either the hip or the core is wobbly and weak, the knee is forced to cope with additional stresses which would otherwise be left to those other regions. The crucial role played by these two elements outside of the knee has only been emphasized in orthopedics and sports medicine in the last ten to fifteen years, but that makes them no less worthy of attention.

Knee stability is not just a matter of ACL strength—other ligaments, the two menisci, articular cartilage, tendons, muscles like the quadriceps and hamstrings, and ultimately the hip and the core are all important components of a complex system which maintains the knee's anatomical integrity. The ACL deserves our focus, however, for its vulnerability to the forces of athletic movements, its poor healing capacity, the consequences of its rupture, and the opportunities that exist to preserve it. It is the perfect target for a prevention strategy.

CHAPTER TWO

The Fragile State of the ACL

NINA WAS THE KIND OF STAR who loved to *play* basketball as much as her friends and family loved to *watch* her play basketball. She was, in a word, spectacular. And, with twelve seconds left in a tight game against her high school's biggest rival, this varsity squad 14-year-old looked poised to do something spectacular, indeed. That's when a hard pivot to avoid a defender produced the "pop" that suggested her biggest fear: Nina had torn her ACL.

But she was not one to despair. A young woman of action and a counterexample to any stereotypes regarding athletes and intellect—her father, a professor at Princeton, had seen to that— Nina did no more than introduce herself before promptly request- ing a "patellar tendon autograft bone-tendon-bone anterior cruciate ligament reconstruction." After examining her knee and MRI, and discussing at length how she planned to use her knee, I had no choice but to agree with her. I hesitate to call any case easy; each patient truly requires attention to her individual aims, attributes, and needs to determine the appropriate course of treat- ment. But this was about as clear-cut as it gets. You'll learn more about surgical options in the next chapter; for now, I will say just that, given Nina's athleticism and athletic goals, I agreed that the operation she named was the one she would get. Prior to going in to the operating room, she decided that she would name her new ACL graft "LeBronna," after LeBron James. She was headed back to the court.

And she got there fast. Looking at Nina's face, you would never guess the intensity that was within. She worked harder than anyone in her rehabilitation to get back to her love, basketball. Her second game of the new season was marked by the brilliance that her fans— none more dedicated than her dad—had remembered from years past. That is, until a fierce plant and cut on the same leg brought with it just what she and her family had feared most. That pop only sounds worse the second time around.

This time, the case was not simple—a revision operation never is. But Nina's unshakable will certainly made it simpler. She wanted to play basketball, and I would do what I could to help her, by using transplanted tissue to reconstruct her ACL a second time. Six months later, only the scars would tell you that Nina had been operated on twice in the same number of seasons. Not quite as effervescent as she was at her first return, she nonetheless grew more impressive by the day. Unfortunately, that trend would be cut short.

I wish that what they say about lightning I could say about young athletes, but, in Nina's case, disaster struck not once, not twice, but *three* times. A misstep in practice had her back in my office, her knee swollen and painful. At first glance, it looked grim. I certainly didn't have to look at Nina's chart to jog my memory of her history. She and her parents had approached her treatment with the same intense, methodical, and deliberate attitude with which Nina had honed her athletic ability. Consultations were extensive, detailed, and exhausting for all involved—we overlooked nothing. This particular visit taxed the four of us more than any before it, because the discussion took a course it never had before: for the first time, we were discussing in earnest the end of Nina's basketball career.

Surgery is draining, both physically and emotionally—for all patients, the less of it, the better. But that wasn't the only reason I suggested a non-operative treatment plan. Perhaps counter-intuitively, it was because Nina's third injury wasn't actually as bad as her first two. My examination of her knee revealed that her ligament was still providing resistance and was not completely torn. The tests that I perform to evaluate the integrity of the ligament were negative. Although the MRI showed some injury to her reconstructed ligament, I believed that Nina had enough tissue left to afford her a life of mobility, without a third surgery. I suggested she consider ending her basketball career, since the risk of further injury was not worth the anguish, in my opinion. There is no right or wrong decision in such cases; it comes down to a patient's own philosophy and desires.

Nina and her family decided to take my advice, but only after much deliberation—ending Nina's basketball career was not something anyone took lightly. But the spectacular player is still leading a spectacular life. She is starting her junior year at Princeton, where Nina studies hard—at least, her father thinks so—and plays hard, joining her friends to play recreational sports and dance. Her knee has remained stable over the five years since she last injured it, and she has been able to live a normal life. Nina's is an all too familiar story and one which defines many of the risk factors associated with ACL tears.

None of Nina's injuries were caused by contact, which is typical of ACL tears. More than two-thirds of all ACL tears are sustained in such "non-contact" situations, many of them occurring during a landing from a jump or cutting or pivoting on the leg. Most of these injuries occur while playing sports, particularly those which rely heavily on the cutting, pivoting, jumping or rapid deceleration just mentioned (i.e., soccer, basketball and volleyball).

Gender also is a contributing factor: Not only are more females playing competitive sports, but, according to many studies, females are as much as six times more likely to tear their ACLs than their male counterparts in these at-risk sports.[29-34] Theories range from hormonal and biomechanical factors to poor neuromuscular control, but the chances of incurring a debilitating knee injury is far greater for females, especially adolescent girls.

These are just some of the associated risk factors related to ACL injuries. In this chapter, I will touch on all of them, including why it is that your son or daughter (or maybe even you) may be in danger of becoming part of this growing and disturbing epidemic.

RISK FACTOR #1

CUTTING AND PIVOTING SPORTS
(NON-CONTACT SITUATIONS)

What causes the ACL to tear in the first place? In most instances, it's not because a giant lineman slammed into the side of the knee, or someone was tripped from behind. Contact injuries like these—whether from sports or a traumatic event like a car accident—are generally not within our power to systematically prevent. But non-contact injuries like Nina's are both eminently preventable and far more common. In fact, most ACL injuries (about 70 percent) occur in non-contact situations, often when the athlete is landing from a jump, planting and cutting sharply to avoid a defender, or coming to an abrupt stop (as to control the ball in soccer or change direction). Take a look at our basketball player Nina, described above. She tore her own ACL and her first reconstruction, without being contacted by anyone else.

In each instance, Nina's knee was put in the at-risk position that I mentioned earlier, which can be defined as fairly straight-legged with the foot remaining planted on the ground and the knee twisted inward (a "knock-kneed" position referred to as "knee valgus"). In this knock-kneed state, the tibia (shinbone) often thrusts forward of the femur (thigh bone), tearing the ACL apart.

Even in a sport like football, which thrives on physical contact, non-contact ACL tears are the norm. The New England Patriots' Wes Welker was enjoying one of the finest seasons for a wide receiver in National Football League history when, in the final game of the 2009 NFL regular season, he went down on just the third play from scrimmage. The smallish receiver had faked going back over the middle and turned in the other direction after catching a short pass from quarterback Tom Brady, himself a victim of a torn ACL. As he turned upfield, Welker tried to juke a defender who stood between him and a possible touchdown. In video replays, Welker's left foot appeared to get caught in the turf as he planted on his left leg, his knee bending so far forward it nearly touched the ground. The defender never laid a hand on him. Welker had torn the ACL and medial collateral ligament in his left knee, ending his season with a league-leading 123 catches. Non-contact injuries occur not only in high school athletes, but also in world class and professional athletes as well.

It is in these dynamic cutting, pivoting, jumping, and tackling sports, such as soccer, basketball, and football, where athletes are most likely to injure their ACL. Other sports, such as handball, volleyball, gymnastics, skiing, and tennis, also leave the knee vulnerable to ACL tears for the same reasons. If you've had previous knee issues, or you want to protect your child from tearing her ACL, sports such as swimming, golf, baseball, and ice hockey offer you a safer athletic arena. In these sports, the non-contact "at-risk" athletic moves with a planted foot either do not occur, or do so much less frequently. It is virtually impossible to tear one's ACL while swimming or golfing and relatively uncommon to do so while playing baseball or ice hockey.

ACL injuries can also occur with other types of trauma, such as a car accident or falling down stairs. A 50-year-old man came to see me with an ACL tear he sustained during a team-building day of events for the bank where he worked as an executive. The employees were teamed up to compete in athletic activities, and, when he landed after jumping over a hurdle, he tore his ACL. The injury can occur outside of the basketball court or soccer field, but the vast majority (nearly 90 percent) occur while participating in sports-related activities.[35]

RISK FACTOR #2

YOUR AGE

Young people, particularly those in their adolescence, tend to sustain more ACL injuries, because they're the most physically active. According to a study by the American Academy of Orthopaedic Surgeons done in 2000, the highest incidence of ACL tears was in individuals 15 to 25 years old who participated in pivoting sports. In an article that I co-authored with my colleague Dr. Stephen Lyman, head of biostatistics at Hospital for Special Surgery, entitled "Epidemiology of Anterior Cruciate Ligament Reconstruction," published in *The Journal of Bone and Joint Surgery*, we found that the highest rate of subsequent ACL reconstruction within one year of the initial ACL surgery was in teenage patients.[36]

On the surface, these numbers seem surprising, based on the growing obesity problem we have with children in America and the explosion of sedentary activities like internet browsing, texting and video games. Yet our nation's youth is taking to the playing fields more than ever before. As I mentioned in the introduction, there are an estimated 41 million kids playing competitive sports today, many of them females, a group which has grown substantially since the passing of Title IX in 1972. If kids are not playing organized sports, then they're jumping rope, shooting baskets on the playground, or playing hide and seek. They're often up on their feet running around, and accidents can lead to injury.

Further, children will often engage in activities that are higher risk than those which adults find entertaining. For example, a 12-year-old patient of mine, Keith Connolly, tore his ACL in a "stair jumping" competition. The kid who jumped the greatest number of stairs was declared the winner. This boy's final jump of 10 stairs won him the awe of his peers, but also landed him on my operating table to have his ACL reconstructed and meniscus repaired.

According to 2003 statistics from the U.S. Consumer Product Safety Commission, children under the age of 15 accounted for more than 3.5 million sports-related injuries in the U.S. that year.

Besides being more active in sports, children also tend to be much more flexible than adults (your ligaments, tendons, and joints lose elasticity as you get older). Because they're so flexible, kids will put their bodies in positions that most adults wouldn't even think of trying. When, for example, was the last time you saw a 50-year-old attempting a backward somersault, handstand, or single-leg split? There's a reason why our U.S. Women's Gymnastics teams are made up of predominantly teenagers and that's because they can tumble, flip, and control their bodies through a wide range of positions.

RISK FACTOR #3

YOUR GENDER

Several studies have shown that female athletes, particularly those in the cutting and pivoting sports (basketball and soccer, primarily) at the high school and college levels are as much as six times more likely to tear their ACLs than their male counterparts competing in the same sports.[29-34] They're also more likely to come back for a subsequent operation on either knee within one year (based on our research mentioned above). Indeed, a good percentage of the patients for whom I perform ACL reconstructions are females from the ages of 12 to 18. The reason for this is unclear, but theories range from hormonal and anatomical differences to poor biomechanics and neuromuscular control.

Poor Biomechanics

According to Dr. Myklebust's research entitled "Injury Mechanisms for Anterior Cruciate Ligament Injuries in Team Handball Players: A Systematic Video Analysis" (published in the *American Journal of Sports Medicine*, 2004),[37] the primary cause of ACL injury appeared to be "a forceful valgus collapse with the knee close to full extension, combined with external or internal rotation of the tibia." The term valgus means knock-kneed—i.e., the knees turned inward to face each other.

Females tend to be born with this valgus condition more commonly than males, putting them at greater risk of being in the "at-risk position" (straight-legged and knock-kneed) for tearing the ACL. When the knee is in this position during a landing from a jump, or from planting the foot while running to pivot on the leg, the ACL is at risk of tearing. Weak hips can also contribute to this increased valgus position. If you land in a straight-legged position on one leg and the hip is weak, the opposing hip tends to drop and, as a result, you have to compensate by becoming even more knock-kneed to keep yourself from falling over.

In the above-mentioned study, a team of medical doctors and coaches studied videotape of ACL injuries among female team handball players over a 12-year period, interviewing many of the victims. They found that most ACL tears occurred in a plant-and-cut faking movement, with the foot planted firmly on the floor and outside the knee. The knee was barely bent at all, and in a valgus position, which caused the ACL to rupture. Several players were also injured when landing on one leg after a jump shot. Once again, the foot was firmly fixed to the floor; the knee was only slightly bent and in valgus, and most of the body weight was on the injured leg. The increasing valgus angle caused the knee to collapse and the ACL to rip apart.

Anatomical

I already touched on one of the bigger anatomical differences between females and males in the previous section—which is increased knee valgus. There are other obvious differences, too, including wider hips in females, greater foot pronation, and a larger Q angle (angle of quadriceps relative to the patellar tendon insertion through the center of the kneecap), but none of these physical differences has been proven to be a precursor for an ACL injury.

A much less obvious anatomical difference between the two genders is the femoral notch, which is the passage at the bottom of the femur (thigh bone) where the ACL attaches to the femur and tibia to cross the knee joint. This tends to be much narrower in women. A smaller notch, some have theorized, could cause the ACL to tear, because there is less room for it.

Another obvious difference between the two sexes is that most females don't carry the muscle mass or strength that males do, and that goes for the lower body as well as the upper body. Since females are typically weaker than males after puberty and show signs of increased flexibility after puberty, it stands to reason that their hamstrings are less powerful. This can lead to less shock absorption upon landing than their male counterparts receive, with more stress transmitted to the ACL.

Hormonal

It's been widely speculated that females are more susceptible to tearing their ACLs just before or after their monthly menstrual period.[4,38,39] Females experience a rapid surge of estrogen just prior to ovulation, usually between days 10 and 14 of the cycle. An increase in estrogen, the primary female sex hormone, can contribute to joint laxity—i.e., looser, less stable joints—and increased flexibility, and have a negative impact on neuromuscular coordination. Nevertheless, it remains unclear if this mechanism has an important role in female ACL injuries.

Too much flexibility can be a bad thing for the ACL. Consider: if someone is double-jointed, he can touch his thumb to his forearm or hyperextend his elbow. Being loose jointed puts you at a higher risk for tearing your ACL, because your knee can get into a position that is at-risk, specifically with the leg relatively straight or hyperextended and the knee in valgus. Landing in such a position could hyperextend the knee even more, putting a tremendous amount of stress on the ACL. Although flexibility increases one's risk for ACL injury, it remains unclear if hormonal changes do. I have certainly treated many young females who have torn their ACLs prior to their first menstrual period and the hormonal surge that goes along with it.

Neuromuscular Coordination

In a study in the *American Journal of Sports Medicine* on plyometric training in female athletes, it was determined that men have three times more knee bend (flexion) than women when decelerating while landing.[40,41] At the same point in time, women not only land with straighter legs, but have increased knee valgus (females land in a more knock-kneed position). The study theorizes that the imbalance in hamstrings-to-quadriceps strength is to blame. Females tend to have stronger quadriceps than hamstrings, creating an unstable environment for the knees. The over-firing of the quads may prevent the female athlete from flexing their knee properly upon landing.

By activating the quadriceps and hamstrings muscles at the same time, one maintains greater joint stability in the knee. The ability to balance oneself better, especially on one leg, is critical to stabilizing the knee joint and avoiding ACL injuries. Therefore, poor proprioception may be another mechanism that leaves women susceptible to ACL tears. Proprioception essentially means having a feel for your body in space, something I will discuss further in Chapter Six. The better you're able to sense where your leg is, and what your muscles are doing, the quicker and more efficient your movements are. If your coordination is slow, you can land improperly and injure yourself.

RISK FACTOR #4

PRIOR ACL RECONSTRUCTION

The risk of subsequent ACL reconstruction surgery on either knee within one year is 1.9 percent, this according to our 2009 *Journal of Bone and Joint Surgery* study.[36] While this doesn't represent a substantial risk, it does mean that if you've torn your ACL before, you are at a higher risk of tearing it again, or of injuring the other knee. Patients who tear their ACL also have a higher risk of requiring further knee surgery and of developing arthritis.

The Multicenter Orthopedic Outcomes Network (MOON) is a group of orthopedic surgeons who began collecting data on our ACL patients ten years ago. In one of our studies, we found that the risk of tearing the ACL graft within two years of surgery was three percent, and the risk of having the other ACL reconstructed in the same time frame was also three percent.[42] People who have torn their ACL once have proven that they are at higher risk, as are their first-degree relatives.[43] The fact that there's a genetic predisposition indicates that the factors above are likely inherited. This indicates that in many cases, ACL tears are more than just bad luck. Later on, I'll discuss other cases that illustrate the genetic factor.

In summary, there are identified risk factors that increase one's chances of tearing an ACL. Although this injury can be fixed, the best option is to never be injured in the first place. The key is to avoid the epidemic. In later chapters, I will explain how this is possible.

CHAPTER THREE

If Your ACL Tears

PREVENTION IS THE GOAL, and the focus of this book, but what if the injury has already occurred? While the old adage that "prevention is the best medicine" is particularly true in the case of the ACL, try telling that to the basketball player who just tore one! Unfortunately, that player's course of action is not at all cut-and-dried. In this chapter, I'll discuss the options open to patients and point to important issues to consider with regard to each one.

The discussion surrounding ACL tears thus far has been almost entirely in relation to sports. There's a good reason for that: the vast majority of ACL tears happen this way.[35,44] People can tear their ACLs without setting foot on a field or court. As I mentioned in the last chapter, the automobile is one culprit; whether that of a passenger or a pedestrian, the ACL can be torn by the forces involved in a car accident. Other traumatic causes include falls from heights and occupational accidents. It's a scary world out there, to be sure, but the athletic arena should scare you the most, if the ACL is what you're worried about.

Many patients who injure their ACL tell the same story. For one thing, the athlete often knows that a particular traumatic event has occurred within the knee. In fact, 70% of the time, the athlete can actually hear or feel a "pop" as the ACL ruptures.[45,46] One wrong pivot is all it takes to tear the ACL on an otherwise uneventful Saturday afternoon; the player will generally hear and feel that characteristic sound. Other classic signs of ACL tear include swelling of the knee within an hour of the injury, and certainly within three hours. This, however, is when the similarities among different patients may end.

There is a huge amount of variability in the way that patients respond to an ACL tear. Naturally, this depends on the severity of the tear itself. But it also depends on the level of mental distraction, associated injuries, and the movements involved in the particular sport being played. Some athletes finish out the game or even play for weeks before experiencing the kinds of symptoms that bring them into the doctor's office. Some, on the other hand, are forced to make it back to the sidelines on one leg, unable even to bear weight on the knee that has been injured.

This variability makes it possible for patients to cause further damage to their knees by returning to sports when they shouldn't. I discussed earlier the relationship between ACL deficiency and arthritis development, via episodes of giving way and meniscal and cartilaginous damage. This possibility makes prevention of the ACL tear even more crucial to preserve the knee as much as possible.

The fact is, as I'll reiterate later on, ACL reconstruction is an established and successful procedure. Of course, that does not mean that every patient needs it—a physician or surgeon experienced in sports medicine can help determine the right course of treatment. Any athlete who hears a pop and experiences swelling in the knee should see a doctor as soon as possible and, in most cases, obtain an MRI as well.

This imaging technology has revolutionized the way we care for knee injuries, offering a level of diagnostic detail that surgeons could only dream of before the advent of MRI.[47] Elements of diagnosis that were once matters of pure guesswork now practically pop off of the screen—if you know what you're looking for. Meniscal tears, loose fragments of bone and cartilage, subtle ligament injuries, and bone bruises—they're all there in high contrast. In fact, the bone bruise had never even been mentioned in a diagnosis before MRI made it visible. Also known as a bone contusion or subchondral fracture, this particular pathology may as well not have existed, for all we knew. And MRI doesn't just help us diagnose accurately; it helps us diagnose quickly. In the first few days after an injury, the knee is often too painful and swollen to yield useful information upon physical examination. But the MRI machine doesn't care how swollen that joint looks from the outside—it will deliver an image of what has happened on the inside.

MRI is most useful, however, in combination with the physical examination, because images can be misleading. There are cases in which the MRI offers a grim outlook—the patient's ACL looks entirely ruptured and useless—when a physical exam indicates that function remains. Conversely, an MRI may indicate an intact ACL that is demonstrated by physical exam to be entirely nonfunctional, and which would turn out to be loose and floppy when probed during subsequent surgery. I have reviewed MRIs that appear to have captured a perfect ACL; meanwhile, the patients complain of instability.

But how could an MRI be *wrong*? It is a veritable picture of what's going on inside the knee, isn't it? The answer has to do with the image properties of scar tissue. While an MRI will never display an intact ACL shortly after an acute ACL injury, chronic ACL deficiency in some cases can be more difficult to identify using this imaging technique. Over time, even a torn ACL can produce scar tissue that, in some cases, creates the appearance of a wholly intact ligament on MRI. Unfortunately, this scar tissue may not provide much in the way of ligamentous function. It is weak and lacks elasticity compared to the original structure. A mere image, however, will not make this distinction. This scenario also highlights the importance of a detailed medical history in making a diagnosis. Events past—and the time elapsed since their occurrence—play an important role.

To find out how well an ACL actually works, a sports medicine specialist needs to examine it. You've probably heard experts, whether doctors or mechanics, say that their extensive experience has imbued them with a certain ineffable sense of the physical matter they know so well, an ability to "get a feel for it" that is "hard to describe." This is not the kind of examination that I mean. There are specific tests which can be performed on the knee to evaluate the functionality of the ACL.

The first is the Lachman test, which requires the physician to bend the knee to twenty or thirty degrees of flexion, then pull forward on the tibia while holding the femur in place. There are two things to look for: the extent of the tibia's forward motion and the firmness of its endpoint. The latter can be described in terms of a rope—imagine holding each end such that the middle hangs slack, then pulling. When the rope reaches full extension, you can feel a characteristic "snap"—the endpoint. The ACL is no different, when it is intact, that is. A torn ACL will have a palpably "soft" endpoint, since its integrity has been compromised, the pulling resisted only by the other soft tissues holding the knee together.

The pivot shift test is another useful diagnostic tool. An ACL-deficient knee will allow the tibia to come forward at full extension, since that ligament would normally restrain this movement. The pivot shift test involves bending the knee back from this fully straight position. Upon reaching approximately twenty degrees of flexion, the iliotibial band—a soft tissue structure on the lateral side of the knee—moves from a position in front of the knee's center of rotation to a position behind it. This pulls the tibia back into place in one swift motion (the "pivot shift") that is easily observed, and which simply will not happen unless the ACL is torn. This shift can be very obviously abnormal, and it indicates that the ACL is not functional. The exception is the rare patient who is loose-jointed and thus has a natural amount of pivot shift. In this scenario, however, the knee in question can simply be compared to the patient's other knee and examined for a greater amount of shift.

The only shortcoming of these physical examinations is their requirement that the patient relax the joint being tested. This is difficult to do with a sore, swollen knee that is fresh from a recent injury, as mentioned earlier when I highlighted the importance of MRI. But testing of the ACL is not the only reason to get a physical examination from a doctor. It is absolutely crucial that the other ligaments of the knee be examined as well. Although MRI is an incredibly useful tool for the care of knee injuries, it cannot always reliably convey the clinical relevance of a ligamentous injury in terms of functionality. And ACL injury management should not go forward without an awareness of the functional status of the ligaments around the ACL.

The reason, as is so often the case in surgical matters, takes us right back to anatomy. Remember that the various ligaments of the knee differ not just in their function but in their capacity to return to form. The medial collateral ligament (MCL)—so commonly injured in conjunction with the ACL—heals much more quickly; ACL reconstructive surgery may be delayed to allow the MCL to repair itself. A more extensive multi-ligament knee injury, however, may have us planning for surgery for even just a few days later.

Complex surgery involving multiple repairs and reconstructions, perhaps to the PCL or posterolateral corner, is often best done early after injury when the surgical dissection is easier and the anatomy easier to define, since scar tissue has not formed yet. If more than one of the ligaments are torn, the knee will almost certainly become unacceptably unstable. In this case, fixing just the ACL won't necessarily solve the problem. In fact, I treated an eighteen-year-old patient whose deficiency in a ligament other than the ACL went ignored for such a long period of time that he had undergone four ACL reconstructions—each of which failed—before I even met him.

Tom Filko was in a bad spot when he arrived in my office, having been in and out of the operating room over the preceding four years with a history that listed almost as many surgeons as surgeries. Tom's four reconstructions had been performed by three different doctors, each in a different location. All of this made me hesitate to operate on Tom's knee. After four failed surgeries on the same joint, the chance of failure on the fifth was not insignificant. But his knee was so unstable with simple daily activities that surgery was the only option if Tom wanted to live a somewhat normal life as an eighteen-year-old.

A closer look at Tom's knee revealed something encouraging. Physical examination pointed to a loose medial collateral ligament that had never been addressed. When surgery for a specific problem fails on multiple successive attempts, the recognition of an associated problem can be cause for celebration. There was work to be done, however, that not all revision cases require.

Each ACL reconstructive surgery leaves tunnels in the femur and tibia, as described in the next chapter on surgical technique. Tom had as many tunnels in his bones as you'd expect of someone who had undergone no less than four reconstructions. Before working on his ligaments, I took Tom to the operating room and filled those tunnels with bone allograft from a cadaver—essentially just minced bone material that would become infused with Tom's own cells and constitute new bone.

Six months later, I operated on the ligaments themselves, to reconstruct both his ACL and MCL. I recommended that he avoid aggressive sports from then on, but, as I'll discuss later, patients often take such suggestions with a grain of salt. How much pick-up basketball he's been playing, I'll never know, although he has admitted to some. But Tom's knee has been stable more than two years and counting, far longer than any of his previous surgeries had done the job. The ACL is only one part of a system, and the other parts—in this case, the MCL—must not be ignored.

Those elements of the knee which are particularly salvageable with early operation also deserve attention. A displaced bucket-handle tear to the meniscus, for example, in which a piece of the meniscus is actually flipped into the space within the knee, like the handle of a bucket, can be stitched back into place if caught early, as is the case with other meniscal tears amenable to repair. Because meniscal repairs have a much higher failure rate if the ACL is deficient, we routinely go ahead and reconstruct the ACL at the same time. Similarly, a piece of loose cartilage in the joint will push us to perform surgery earlier—as surgery is the only way to address the problem—at which point we would usually reconstruct the ACL as well.

Despite the importance of an accurate assessment of the ACL and the number of tools with which the physician can determine it, the raw physical state of an ACL injury is not the only factor in choosing how to treat a patient. What matters most is how they live their lives. Activity level is paramount. A patient for whom cutting and pivoting is a way of life—basketball and soccer players—and who wants to get back out there and keep doing it, requires a different sort of treatment than the patient whose tear is identical to that of the athlete, but who doesn't participate in any sports that involve cutting and pivoting.

It is well documented that highly active ACL-injured patients who engage in cutting and pivoting movements will have a high risk of experiencing knee instability if they don't have ACL reconstruction.[48-50] Is there a chance that non-operative treatment will succeed in such an active patient? Of course there is. But the chance is a small one, and it comes at a cost.

On average, it can take three months, six months, or even longer until that patient can take to the field again after non-operative treatment for an ACL injury. All the while, instability—and the operation that should have come earlier—is practically inevitable. Why rehabilitate twice? And even if rehabilitation time were a non-issue, there is another concern more deserving of our attention: arthritis. As explained by Dr. Bruce Levy from the Mayo Clinic in the *New England Journal of Medicine*, a return to aggressive cutting and pivoting sports has a very high risk of failure, and that patient will most likely experience the kind of recurrent giving way in the knee that limits sports participation, damages the meniscus and cartilage and leaves arthritis in its wake.[50] That patient ought to undergo ACL reconstruction.

But not every patient wants to do tomorrow—and the next day, and every weekend—what landed her in the clinic today. If cutting and pivoting sports are no longer on the agenda, we may elect to rehabilitate that patient without surgery. This is generally a better option for older patients who are more likely to accept a less active lifestyle, or for a lawyer or teacher who is relatively sedentary. If the instability is minor and occasional, the patient may simply elect to live with that limitation, alter lifestyle, and cope.

I did mention earlier, however, that, as the years go on, patients are staying active—and more aggressively active—into their later years. Because fifty-three-year-old competitive tennis players are no longer rare, age is no longer a firm determinant of treatment. What it really comes down to is the amount and kind of physical activity in which the patient aims to engage. Keep in mind that this activity need not fall in the sporting category. For example, if someone needs to be able to cut and pivot for their job, they should have reconstructive surgery. Neither a police officer nor a firefighter will be allowed to return to active duty with an ACL-deficient knee, since a giving way episode at a crucial moment could mean the difference between life and death, not just for them, but for their partners or the civilians they protect.

It is the pediatric patient whose age and activity level more often create a dilemma. On the one hand, ACL reconstructive surgery can damage the growth plates on the ends of the tibia and femur that comprise the knee.[51-53] Naturally, it is desirable neither to reduce one leg's capacity to grow nor alter its geometry relative to that of the other leg. On the other hand, it is exceedingly difficult to change the activity level of a child. Try asking young

Bobby to stop tearing around the school yard with his friends, and see where that gets you. As mentioned earlier, young and highly active ACL-deficient patients will generally experience the kind of instability that damages meniscus and cartilage and brings with it the possibility of arthritis later on. Indeed, recurrent instability in children has a poor prognosis; more often than not, they will damage these tissues if the ACL is not reconstructed.[54,55] For this reason, and because there are effective techniques to avoid growth plate damage in pediatric patients, I have performed reconstructive surgery on countless young patients with ACL tears with excellent results.

Regardless of patient age, however, the question is not always a simple yes or no to surgery. Sometimes, the best course of action is to wait and see. Many patients for whom the decision is difficult end up doing just fine with non-operative care, while others will eventually undergo ACL reconstruction even years after the injury. If they develop instability at any point and are dissatisfied with their quality of life due to that sense of instability and lack of trust in the knee, they can always elect to have surgery at that point. In fact, I have found that patients who have the surgery later are often among my happiest patients. Unlike an ACL patient who has surgery soon after the injury and returns to all sports following the operation, as expected, these people have had their knee give way repeatedly. They are then overjoyed to have that problem go away. Unfortunately, they are at higher risk of having cartilage and meniscus damage at the time of surgery.[56,57]

The risk of non-operative care is the instability that can lead to meniscal and cartilaginous damage, which can be both painful by itself and lead to arthritis down the line. Whether surgery categorically prevents arthritis is a matter of great controversy, but surgery can eliminate the instability that puts the other tissues at risk, which in turn leads to arthritis.[58,59]

Of course, surgery is not without its own set of risks, which I discuss with every patient who considers it. Many of these risks are unique neither to ACL reconstruction nor to orthopedic surgery in general. Anesthesia, for one, can bring with it complications, but these are minimized by two factors: the relative good health of the patients who typically undergo this type of surgery and the use of regional, rather than general, anesthesia. Infection is always a risk as well, though, typically, antibiotics and, in the rare case, further surgery will take care of the problem. Blood clots are possible, though I do not use blood thinners unless the patient has a family or personal history of clots.[60-62] The fear, of course, is that a blood clot could turn into a pulmonary embolism, which can be devastating. The scientific data show, however, that blood clots among the population undergoing ACL reconstruction are exceedingly rare.[60]

More specific risks of ACL reconstruction include the possibility of severing nerve tissue or damaging a blood vessel, though the latter two are exceptionally uncommon; I have witnessed neither. Pain and stiffness in the joint are normal after this kind of surgery but usually fade with time, though some patients will continue to experience these symptoms and must receive treatment to address them.

The most obvious risk of ACL reconstruction is that the patient can tear the new ligament. Regardless of the source, grafts are not infallible, with a 5–10% failure rate on average.[63] I must emphasize here the distinction between the average and the individual. Certain patients are far more likely to tear the graft than others; credit differences in age, graft type, and, above all else, activity level. A teenage female basketball player will find herself at a risk greater than 10% if she continues to play competitively enough, often enough, for long enough. Lottery tickets don't often justify the initial outlay, but if you purchase three hundred tickets every day for ten years, well, you just might hit the jackpot. The kids who are playing on multiple teams, year round in high-risk sports are at the highest risk. Older patients who play cutting and pivoting sports only occasionally are, of course, at much lower risk.

Outcomes after ACL reconstruction are no different, and, as with the kind of gambling just mentioned, there are different games with different odds. In basketball, the odds are stacked in your favor, but you won't like what's in the pot. Simply put, I believe that activity level is the single biggest factor in determining a patient's risk of re-injury after ACL reconstruction. Despite the relative rarity of ACL graft tears, if patients engage in high-risk sporting activities with enough frequency, their risk increases dramatically. If they tore their own ACL during sports, they can certainly tear the graft.

Should patients retire from sports after tearing their ACL? Lifestyle modification is a complex matter, and the best course of action is rarely crystal clear. The issue gets us thinking about the goals of healthcare in general, even considering deeper philosophical questions with which we've all grappled. Is the body to be preserved for its own sake or used to greatest effect? Is it an end or a means? Eat the cheeseburger and fries; life is short! But do the cheeseburger and fries have the potential to shorten life enough that it just isn't worth it?

Suffice it to say that the matter of returning to sports is one that must be addressed on an individual basis and with great care. If the female basketball player just mentioned does in fact tear her graft and then re-tears a second, or the ACL in her other knee, it may be time to pursue another sport. As I described in Chapter Two, Nina O'Connor decided to do just that, but not before enduring a treatment rollercoaster that mixed soaring hope with crushing disappointment.

PERSONAL HISTORY ISN'T THE ONLY KIND that matters, though. Family history can be just as important in considering the risk of ACL injury. It could be more than a family can collectively bear, to send two soccer-playing daughters back to the field after each of them has torn her ACL, as the Morgans unfortunately had to decide. This could also indicate a genetic predisposition to ACL tears.

There are three charts filed in my office labeled with the surname, "Townsend," and I do not believe that it's a coincidence. The first I treated was Steph, whose torn ACL I reconstructed successfully when she was fifteen. It looked like a happy ending for the Townsends, until Steph's younger sister, Amy, came in with the same injury when she was only twelve. This was particularly difficult for the family, as another year of recovery for them was a lot to take. Nevertheless, the risk of knee injury without the surgery was higher in the long run.

Despite that, Mrs. Townsend had no desire to send her daughter into the operating room. I would not typically treat a patient like

Amy with non-operative care, so mom wasn't getting her advice from me. She based her decision on her own experience: she had been living normally for years without a single intact ACL. When she told me of her own injuries, my examination revealed bilateral, asymptomatic ACL tears in this mother of the two daughters, each of whom had torn her ACL at a young age. When it came to Amy's treatment plan, Mrs. Townsend had the last word. So far, Amy has been fine, playing sports with her peers and generally just ignoring the problem. While this scenario is uncommon, there are patients who can function in sports without their ACL, but they are the exception to the rule. For each one of these, there are many, many more who have returned to sports without their ACL and gone on to have recurrent instability with meniscal and cartilage damage. Nevertheless, I relate this bittersweet anecdote to make a couple of points about ACL injury.

For one, you're more likely to tear this ligament if a sibling or parent has done the same.[43] I've tried to convey this message adequately to my good friend, David Konay, himself an ACL reconstruction patient whose wife has had *both* of her ACLs reconstructed, one of which tore again and needed to be revised. Where is David's son? He's probably on the soccer field right now. For a kid who can count a total of four ACL reconstructions between his two parents, soccer may not be the best choice!

I tell the Townsends' story also to point out that an ACL tear may have practically no effect on the patient's lifestyle. Just ask Ellen or Amy, at least so far. Some patients can carry on without ACL function and not even tear a meniscus. That said, my own experience in combination with available research leads me to believe that, if she continues with high level sports, she has a high chance of developing instability in the future.[48,64]

Then again, this story is not one that you'll hear often; more than 90% of patients who tear their ACL end up with a knee that is too unstable to play aggressive cutting and pivoting sports. As I discussed earlier, this puts the meniscus and cartilage at risk—after that, arthritis may be only a matter of time. Generally, a patient has torn his ACL doing something he loves. When you love to do something, you want to keep doing it, and although in medicine and surgery there are always exceptions, the risks of returning to cutting and pivoting sports without an ACL outweigh the benefits.

But if the last chair you sat on before you heard that pop was hanging from a cable, listen up: skiers may buck the trend. I'm about to describe a subset of patients that is still relatively small, but they exhibit a recovery pattern that has practical implications for those with a similar mechanism of injury. The skiers to whom I refer are typically over thirty and come to see me after a low-energy, low-speed fall has ended their day on the slopes. Physical examination and MRI both point to an ACL tear—so far, there's nothing out of the ordinary to report here.

The interesting part happens about 6–8 weeks later, when the physical exam leaves me with eyebrows raised—because the ACL is no longer loose. In the majority of cases, skiers included, the ACL would not have healed in at this point. The topic of conversation would shift to surgery, if their desired activity level suggested it. But there is something about these low-energy skiing injuries that, in some cases, allows the ACL to heal effectively on its own. I said before that the ACL can't heal. While that is generally true, this particular type of injury in lower level skiers is sometimes characterized by unique attributes that allows the ACL to heal enough to maintain stability.

In some of these cases, however, the tear has usually occurred at the point where the ACL attaches to the femur. Rather than a violent tear right through the middle of the ligament—think scissors to the center of a stretched out rubber band—the ACL has been pulled off of the femur, though not very far—think Velcro shoe strap half undone. Because the damage to the ligament is not as extensive, and because the ligamentous tissue is still close to a solid point of attachment, scar tissue can do a decent job of filling in the gap to restore ACL function. While certainly few in number, these particular patients have something to teach us: don't book your surgery as soon as you get to the bottom of the mountain. If you give it six weeks, you just might avoid the knife.

Luckily, we generally wait at least four weeks before operating in any case. In fact, it's not uncommon to wait six weeks before surgery. Operating on a knee that is still swollen and stiff from the injury carries with it a much higher risk of arthrofibrosis, or build-up of scar tissue inside the joint.[114] Injury puts the knee in a particular biologic state. Filled with blood and biochemical mediators of inflammation and healing, the environment is highly responsive to further trauma. In a stiff, painful and swollen knee, the response can come in the form of massive scarring that's not limited to the injured ligament, what we call a "global" response. Like the quadriceps inhibition pathway I'll discuss in relation to rehab, it's an evolutionary mechanism that makes sense on the level of survival: relentless trauma ought to ramp up the production of scar tissue to patch up the wounds.

But all of that scar tissue can turn run-of-the-mill stiffness post-injury into debilitating stiffness for a lifetime, and it's extremely difficult to fix. Stiffness after surgery was not uncommon back in the dark ages of ACL reconstruction, when surgery was often performed right after the injury. But a better understanding of the biology behind the healing process and less invasive surgery has largely done away with the problem. We won't subject the knee to the trauma of surgery before the swelling has resolved and the knee has recovered its full range of motion. I will go so far as to cancel a surgery for this reason alone.

Sam Griswold found this out the hard way after, I suspect, forgoing the use of crutches for those four intervening weeks. I had made clear to Sam that he was not to walk without crutches, nor to limp on the injured knee. Sam could move his knee from five degrees to ninety degrees of flexion (moving the leg from slightly bent to L-shaped) when I first examined him after his ACL had torn. Four weeks later, ready for surgery, Sam could only flex his knee between ten and forty degrees. Although the operating room was ready with my staff and the equipment set up and ready to go, I cancelled his surgery then and there. ACL reconstruction is an elective procedure that can be postponed for another few weeks without increasing risk to the patient. Indeed, the risk of severe stiffness would decrease in this case since he would return a month later with almost no swelling and full motion.

However long a patient waits before ACL reconstruction, they ought to exercise care in choosing the person for the job. And in my line of work, practice makes perfect. Recommendations from friends, family members, and other medical professionals certainly help, but the simple truth is that high-volume surgeons see better outcomes in their patients.[36] This holds not just for orthopedic surgeons but for surgeons in every specialty, and the scientific data proves it.[65-72] If you do a lot of cutting and sewing, you're going to get better at cutting and sewing.

Despite its ubiquity, ACL reconstruction is a complex and technically demanding procedure with many steps. Repetition is completely necessary, if not entirely sufficient, for mastery. Indeed, it was the busiest surgeons who I considered the best and emulated during my own training. It is why I perform ACL reconstruction frequently. Pilots have to stay current; why shouldn't surgeons? Reading, writing, and talking about surgery will not make anyone a better surgeon. You've got to do it.

CHAPTER FOUR

Surgical Treatments

I'VE DESCRIBED ACL RECONSTRUCTION AS COMPLEX and technically demanding. In this chapter, I'll explain what I mean by that, focusing on the choices to be made in connection to this particular procedure. Just as ACL injury treatment is not a simple question of surgery or not, the surgery itself is not the same for all comers.

Part of the reason can be found in the name of the surgery: "reconstruction." This is not a synonym for "repair," but rather refers to a specific type of procedure. To repair a ligament is to sew its two ends back together—simple enough. But to reconstruct it is to actually rebuild the entire ligament using tissue from another source—essentially, to make a new one.

Because of the poor healing capacity of the ACL, repairs don't work predictably. Sutures are not enough to hold this ligament together over a long period of time. That the ACL is generally incapable of such healing was evidenced by the outcomes of repairs in the early days of ACL surgery; fully half of them failed.[73] While repair can be considered in very rare circumstances, reconstruction is overwhelmingly favored, and repair is unpredictable even in those rare circumstances.

Reconstruction presents a question, then: where should the tissue for the new ACL come from? The answer, as with so many of the questions surrounding ACL injury treatment, depends largely on the patient's age, surgical history, and activity level. The options include patellar tendon, quadriceps tendon, and hamstrings from the patient's own knee—referred to as "autograft" tissue—as well as "allograft" tissue sourced from a donor (i.e., cadaver).

Graft source selection is one of the most controversial aspects of ACL reconstruction. A cursory glance at the literature will reveal proponents of every type. Though the point is certainly debatable, the best available evidence supports the use of patellar tendon autograft for high-risk patients if possible. Dr. Iftach Hetsroni, an Israeli surgeon who worked as a fellow with me at the Hospital for Special

Surgery in New York for a year, performed a systematic review of the best studies in the scientific literature—randomized trials that followed up at least 80% of the patients enrolled at a minimum of two years—that address this very question. He found that the failure rate for patellar tendon autograft was roughly 7% and more than twice that for hamstring autografts.[63] My own clinical experience corroborates these findings.

That does not mean, however, that patellar tendon autograft ought to be used in all cases. Remember the importance of activity level: a forty-year-old recreational tennis player is at far lower risk of graft tear than a highly competitive fifteen-year-old midfielder on the soccer team. It is also the fifteen-year-old who can typically bounce right back from the harvesting of a segment of patellar tendon, whereas the forty-year-old could experience a little more difficulty and require more time to rehabilitate. Patellar tendon autograft tissue is removed with a piece of bone from the patella and tibia to which it is attached, making the harvesting procedure more challenging to recover from. This can lengthen the recovery period for older, less conditioned individuals but is much less of a factor for younger and more muscular patients.

Older patients usually have more demands on their time and fewer on their muscles—with a job and a family, rehabilitation is difficult. In cases of lower activity level and older age, I typically recommend using the patient's hamstring or allograft tissue rather than the patellar tendon. While the notion that patellar tendon autograft harvesting inevitably causes insurmountable anterior knee pain is commonly held, this is simply not true in most cases, especially among young patients who simply recover muscle more quickly. On the other hand, it is reasonable to avoid the increased risk of such pain in a patient whose activity level does not require the enhanced graft durability.

Sourcing the graft from a donor is even less invasive, but there are drawbacks. Studies have shown that allograft tissue can be unpredictable, particularly in young, active patients.[74] I only use tissue from a vendor whose processing techniques are familiar to me, but, even then, it's possible that this processing will have unknown effects and that variability can still occur among different donors. These concerns just don't exist when using the patient's own tissue.

Even so, there are cases in which allograft tissue is the best option. When performing revision surgery or a multiligament reconstruction, there are simply fewer graft options. The revision patient may have had patellar tendon or hamstring harvested from the injured knee during the previous surgery; and the multiligament patient simply requires more grafts than would be desirable to harvest from the patient's own body, whatever the location. I frequently use allograft tissue in these situations. As mentioned earlier, patients who are over forty and not participating in aggressive sports are also good candidates for allograft reconstruction in many cases.

The source of the graft, however, is not the only controversial decision. Over the past ten years, research has shown that it may be better to reconstruct both "bundles" of the ACL.[75-77] The ACL is actually made up of two parts, an anteromedial part and a posterolateral part.[78] While this makes sense in theory and even in the laboratory, I don't think it is a good idea for a patient. To accomplish this type of reconstruction, two holes must be created in each bone instead of one. This makes an already complicated operation much more so. It also turns the tibia and femur into Swiss cheese, and, if revision surgery is needed, it is far more difficult to perform. As well, the results to date show little or no difference between "single bundle" and "double bundle" reconstruction.[79-82] So, until we find that two bundles are better than one, we should keep it simple and do what we know works well.

In the end, there are pros and cons to every type of graft for ACL reconstruction, and I review all of these with each patient prior to surgery. Even the aforementioned hamstring autograft can occasionally result in weakness in deep flexion of the knee. There are those who support the use of contralateral patellar tendon—that is, patellar tendon from the patient's uninjured knee.[83,84] This accelerates recovery time in the ACL-injured knee, as it must endure just half of the typical operation; harvesting of the graft is often more painful than the reconstruction itself! But the patient then requires recovery time in the knee which would have been left perfectly intact. Sending a patient home with a bandage on each knee to save a month of recovery time is, in my opinion, not worth it.

Here again, however, the matter is not that simple. If a football player tears his graft and elects to undergo revision reconstruction, only to return yet again to the field, I would most likely harvest patellar tendon from his uninjured knee for the same reason I took that tissue from his injured knee when performing the primary reconstruction. It's the most resilient tissue, and that is precisely what that patient needs. That is exactly what I did for Tom Benson, the starting running back from a local Pennsylvania college. After tearing the patellar tendon graft used by his team physician, I felt his best option to return safely to his sport was to use the same graft from the other knee. I offer these examples to illustrate that there are no standard prescriptions when treating an ACL tear, and graft choice is no exception.

O NCE THE GRAFT SOURCE AND OTHER PARAMETERS are determined, reconstruction can commence. The surgery is done arthroscopically, which means that two small holes are made in the front of the knee, one for the instruments and one for the scope. The scope allows the surgeon to view the inside of the knee in great detail on a TV screen in the operating room. The instruments can remove or

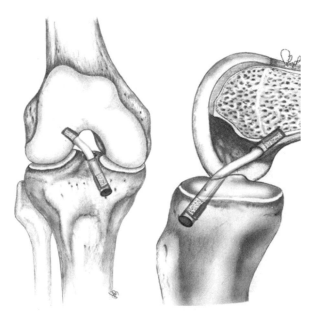

Source: Zaffagnini S, Bruni D, Muccioli GMM, Bonanzinga T, Lopomo N, Bignozzi S, Marcacci M. Single bundle patellar tendon versus non-anatomical double-bundle hamstrings ACL reconstruction: a prospective randomized study at 8 year minimum follow-up. *Knee Surgery, Sports Traumatology, Arthroscopy*, 19(3): 390–397, 2011.

repair torn menisci and are also used to reconstruct the ACL. The surgeon will create tunnels in the tibia and femur such that the graft can be passed through the tibia, across the knee joint, and into the femur. Tunnels are drilled either through a new incision, in the case of an allograft reconstruction, or through the harvest incision, if the patient's patellar tendon or hamstring tissue is being used. The graft is then secured in both the tibia and femur using any one of a number of different types of fixation devices. These include buttons, staples, and screws, and are chosen depending on the type of graft employed. Interference screws, for example, are typically used to secure a patellar tendon graft in the tunnels. These screws are named such because they are squeezed in between the graft and the wall of the tunnel, "interfering" with potential movement between the tissues.

To fixate a hamstring graft, a button is often secured to the end of the graft and pulled back against the end of the outside of the femur bone to hold the graft in place. As with grafts, virtually every combination of fixation devices and methods will find an advocate

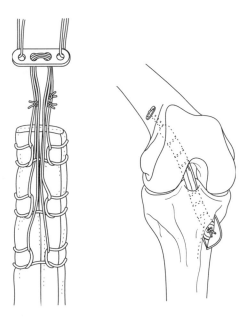

Source: Barrett GR, Papendick L, Miller C. Endobutton Button Endoscopic Fixation Technique in ACL Reconstruction. *Arthroscopy: The Journal of Arthroscopic and Related Surgery.* 11(3): 340–343, 1995.

in one surgeon or another. While there is more evidence to support the use of some than others, there is no categorical right answer. Fixation, like almost every other matter in ACL treatment or in patient care in general, must be considered on a case-by-case basis.

There is one issue, however, which deserves our focus, and to which certain generalizations do apply. The broad overview of ACL reconstruction offered thus far—select a graft, drill tunnels in the correct anatomic location, and secure it well—ignores the more subtle techniques that we apply to an important subset of patients: those who are still growing. I've described ACL injury as an epidemic among young athletes, many of whom have yet to reach their full height when they hear that pop. I would be remiss if I didn't discuss the methods that have been developed to avoid damage to the growth plates of skeletally immature individuals who require ACL reconstruction.

To appreciate the techniques, you need to understand the problem. Damaging a growth plate does not just make the injured leg shorter than the other one; it can alter the alignment of that leg itself. The deformity usually occurs in the lateral region of the distal femur, the end that forms part of the knee joint. The reason is simple: this is where the femoral tunnel is drilled. As the femur continues to grow on the medial side, the leg can bend into a knock-kneed position if the femur is not growing on the lateral side.

The growth plate on the proximal tibia, which rests against the distal femur to form the knee joint, is also vulnerable. The tibial tubercle apophysis (growth plate), located on the anterior region of the tibia where the patellar tendon finds its point of attachment, can be damaged not just by drilling nearby but by a heavily tensioned ACL graft. In such cases, the posterior region of the knee continues to grow, pushing the knee into *recurvatum*, or a hyper-extended position. As you can imagine, either deformity can be devastating to a young athlete's development, not just in terms of sporting ability, but in terms of overall mobility.

The younger the patient is, the bigger the risks he faces; more inches left to grow means more degrees remain to shift away from natural skeletal alignment. Luckily, there is a proven reconstructive technique that obviates the need to drill tunnels through the growth plates.[85-87] It involves the use of a segment of the iliotibial band, mentioned earlier in relation to the pivot shift test, which I route through the knee and around the bones. The graft is anchored with sutures rather than metal hardware. Because the consequences of damage to the growth plates can be severe for a patient with many years of growth remaining, this is the usual method I employ when operating on very young patients.

However, drilling across the growth plates in pediatric patients approaching the end of their growth, usually boys aged 13–15 and girls 12–14, can be safely accomplished if proper technique is employed.[88-90] For one, I always use soft tissue ACL grafts; putting bone across a growth plate, as in a patellar tendon autograft, will halt its development. No less important, I fixate the graft away from the growth plate; metal hardware across the growth plate has an effect similar to that of bone. The third measure is intuitive: I drill small tunnels. Patients at these ages generally furnish relatively small hamstring autografts which require no more than a 6 to 8 mm tunnel through which to pass. It has been shown that, using these methods, we can drill across the growth plates safely.[90]

Beyond the pediatric, there are other issues that are common enough to deserve mention in any discussion of surgical treatment for ACL tear. One of these is the associated meniscal tear. We try to preserve the meniscus, since it is a shock absorber that prevents excessive load on cartilage and therefore delays or prevents arthritis. Our options for a torn meniscus are threefold: do nothing, remove the torn bits, or stitch it together. If it is a very small tear, in some cases we can ignore it and leave it alone. If the tear is larger, however, it will cause pain by getting stuck in the joint and pulling on the capsule of the knee, which has a great deal of nerves and is very sensitive. In such cases, we can remove the torn part, which allows the patient to rehabilitate at the same pace as a regular ACL reconstruction. But, since the meniscus has a job as a shock absorber, if it is a large tear with good blood supply, we prefer to repair and preserve it if possible.

This is more important in young people, since arthritis usually takes a decade or two to begin following meniscus removal, so they have more time for the arthritis to set in. Even if the arthritis becomes very severe, a seventy-year-old patient may elect to have a knee replacement to improve their ability to walk and function.

But a knee replacement is a far less attractive option for a forty-year-old, because these implants are not designed for running or sports. Additionally, knee replacements can loosen over time, and young patients are more likely to have this occur due to their activity and the fact that they have more years to look forward to after the surgery. So, the bottom line is: save the meniscus if you can!

Meniscal repairs usually heal. About eighty percent do well, based on our research,[91] although each case is different based on the tear type, tissue quality and the age of the patient. If the tear is at the outside part of the meniscus, near the capsule of the knee, it has a better blood supply and therefore a better chance to heal. If the tissue is shredded and beaten up like wet Kleenex, it won't heal if you suture it. On the other hand, if it is a clean rip through good, solid tissue, your chances of success will be high. Lateral meniscal tears generally heal better than medial tears, since the blood supply to the lateral meniscus is superior. Lastly, younger patients have higher rates of healing, because their menisci are less degenerative and have better blood supply than those of older patients.[92]

The meniscus, however, is not the only part of the knee that might tear along with the ACL. Other times, one or more other ligaments are torn as well.[93-96] These complex injuries are termed multi-ligament knee injuries, and, in some cases, they may constitute complete knee dislocations, where the end of the thigh bone disassociates from the lower leg bone. These situations usually occur in the setting of major trauma, such as a car accident or a fall from a height, but they can also occur in sports. Because the injury is so severe, the major nerves and arteries in the leg may be damaged, with devastating consequences.

Multi-ligament knee injuries generally require much more extensive surgery, and the rehabilitation is much slower for these patients. Allograft tissue is usually used, because multiple grafts are needed (one for each ligament). Along with my colleagues, I have developed and published techniques to reconstruct the medial and lateral ligament complexes.[20,97] The ability to handle these injuries should be in the armamentarium of all knee ligament surgeons. Fortunately, many patients with these extremely complex injuries can return to their usual activities, including sports in some cases.

REGARDLESS OF THE AGE, ASSOCIATED INJURIES, or activity level of the patient who elects to undergo ACL reconstruction, it is a very successful procedure that must be tailored carefully to that individual. The factors that may make all the difference in surgery— graft source, fixation hardware, tunnel location—are too numerous to list here. But the outcome is usually a good one; patients can move the way they want to and, hopefully, avoid the arthritis that can develop from recurrent knee instability.

On more occasions than I would like to recount, I've stood in exam rooms filled with tears. I don't usually have to tell a patient that her ACL is torn, because she already knows. She has come to me with MRI in hand, because she wants me to perform the surgery. Now and then, however, I am the bearer of bad news. No, not just bad news—*devastating* news. I really do mean that. For many of the people reading this book, this will sound obvious. And the rest may never truly understand my point. But sports is an arena that inspires passion at least equal to that we see in the arts or spheres of intellect. And with the tearing of an ACL, a season is over, and possibly the next, and possibly every one that would have followed. It's why my tears almost flow to join the others'.

Sarah Bricker knew exactly what the term "ACL" means. By her junior year soccer season, how could she not? No less than three of her teammates—Jen, Christina, and Monica—had already torn it. Christina was lucky; the pivot that sent her to the sidelines was born of the intensity that only a championship game can produce. She had torn her ACL at the end of the previous season, and that meant time to recover before the next one. The intensity that had led to her injury also characterized her rehabilitation—Christina never planned to miss a game that next season, which had turned out to be one of her best yet.

Jen knew this all too well, as she had witnessed her friend's startling progress largely from the bench. Having torn her ACL a few months after Christina had, Jen's recovery was progressing slowly, and she found motivation in Christina's progress. Monica's injury was even more recent, and she was still on crutches, watching from the sidelines.

It may seem strange, then, that Sarah was smiling as she waited to see me about her recent knee injury. Although, if your ACL isn't torn, why not smile? Sarah considered herself something of an expert on ACL injury, and this expert had observed in herself neither the overwhelming swelling nor extensive pain that all three of her companions had exhibited in the days that followed their injuries. After performing the Lachman test and taking a look at her MRI, however, I had no doubt that Sarah's ACL was torn. She'd be hearing it from me first.

"How will I get back to playing with my team?" Sarah seemed to pose the question not to me, but to her injured knee, as she stared at it with a mixture of frustration and despair. It is at this moment that one thing becomes quite clear to anyone there to witness it: passion for sports involves so much more than the physical act itself. Athletics are a framework in which vital elements of life develop and find meaning. For many young people, athletics are *the* framework. Years of early-morning practices, team cookouts, and car rides with their daughter to travel games far and wide had already made it clear to Regina and Mike Bricker that Sarah was one of those young people. And I would challenge anyone who knew what they knew, to dismiss as melodrama the sight of mother, father, and daughter in tears, as Sarah uttered the simple statement, "My life is over."

But Memorial Sloan-Kettering Cancer Center is across the street. Teenagers there receive treatment for problems that affect not just a framework into which fit the elements of a good life, but their life itself. Their diseases may shake the very foundations of their lives in ways that a sports injury just won't. More importantly, some of their problems have no true solution. When these kids state what Sarah did, they mean it literally.

ACL injury has a solution in the form of reconstruction. While it may not be infallible, it offers for many the opportunity to engage for the rest of their lives in the athletic pursuit they truly love and, if not that, at least a life of satisfying mobility. At the risk of trivializing injuries like Sarah's, I point this out to the family whose sobbing I fully understand. I gently remind them that it could be worse. Their child will return to an active lifestyle; for that, we can be thankful.

CHAPTER FIVE

Returning Back to Action

UNFORTUNATELY, ACL RECONSTRUCTION REQUIRES more than just a durable graft to achieve a good outcome. Time and discipline are what truly produce a happy ACL-reconstructed patient. Rehabilitation is crucial to success. Surgery is easy for patients—they're sedated or asleep—but what comes after can be quite challenging. Non-operative care, too, delivers results only after months of dedication. In this chapter, I'll explain what patients can expect of the rehabilitation process, whether their treatment involves surgery or not.

Rehabilitation can only be described in somewhat broad terms; it is characterized as much by the tremendous variability observed among patients as by any generalizations we can draw. This is particularly true of non-operative rehab. Without an operation, the starting point is the moment after traumatic injury, descriptions of which will sound quite different depending on whom you ask: "Something sure didn't feel right during those last three shots on goal" indicates a state of affairs quite different from that of the patient who asks, "Can I get some help standing up here?" However, rarely are athletes able to finish the game, nor are they typically on crutches for more than a month to six weeks after the injury.

More common is the patient whose experience is somewhere in between. People usually have trouble walking for a few weeks, and time spent on crutches can range from a few days to several weeks. Patients will typically be able to walk normally within four weeks after the injury. The return to cutting and pivoting sports is another matter entirely and will only rarely happen before three months have passed if they elect to avoid surgery, which is usually not recommended.[50]

A well-designed rehabilitation program is helpful to anyone recovering from an ACL injury. Braces can supplement the rehab work, particularly if there is an associated MCL tear. The brace protects the MCL and allows it to heal over the first month or two following the injury. An ACL brace can offer the same sense of security and stability that even a simple rubber sleeve provides, but with an added degree of mechanical support.

But neither a rehab program nor a brace is a substitute for surgery when the patient sets her sights on cutting and pivoting sports. There is no way to achieve the benefits of a functional ACL without putting a new one in the knee.[49] The brace, however, can play a role after surgery, although this is just as controversial. Part of that controversy stems from the lack of scientific data to support the use of a brace for patients after surgery.[98]

That is, ACL re-injury following surgery is relatively rare. If you follow one hundred ACL reconstruction patients for two years to see how they do after surgery, half of whom wear braces and half of whom do not, you may see as few as two graft tears in the entire study! This is hardly a sound basis on which to draw any conclusion at all, regardless of the group which saw fewer tears. For most patients, I don't recommend a brace after surgery. Nonetheless, I suggest that very-high-risk patients like teenage basketball and soccer players use a brace for a year or two after surgery. Although there is no scientific evidence to support brace use after surgery, there is little downside. The only downsides involve slight discomfort and ergonomic awkwardness. The brace offers some degree of support; when you're at risk, shouldn't you use every tool in the orthopedic arsenal? Since they may benefit the patient, I often use them in cases where risk is the greatest, and the brace therefore offers the highest relative advantage.

However surgeons feel about braces, they will all agree on this: surgery is useless if not followed by a well-executed rehabilitation program. Let it settle down, regain strength, return to sport activities, and regain confidence. These are the things that need to happen before taking a new ACL back to the court or field.

Swelling—it's what keeps a knee from moving the way it should, from returning to the way it was. Swelling prevents the quadriceps from getting stronger as part of a mechanism I'll discuss later on in the chapter, and quadriceps strength is crucial to regaining knee stability for sporting activities. Cryotherapy, or cold therapy, is the age-old treatment for swelling. Devices are commercially available which will circulate water around the knee at a temperature just above freezing. Pumps and compressors do the job formerly accomplished by bags of ice on paper towels. Then again, ice still works, too—thirty minutes on, thirty minutes off.

The strengthening and flexibility afforded by reduced swelling is considered crucial today in a way that it wasn't thirty years ago. Back then, the knee was immobilized in a cast for six weeks after reconstructing the ACL. It eventually became clear that the reconstruction is strong enough to tolerate knee movement right after surgery. My current protocol is for patients to leave the hospital in a brace that keeps the knee locked in a fully extended position. This allows the knee to settle down and the discomfort to subside. After five days of bracing and cryotherapy, I take off the brace and encourage the patient to regain full range of motion. Continuous passive motion machines have been proven to be not necessary and most patients dislike using them.[99] While I also suggest that they bear weight on the knee as much as they can tolerate it, I do not recommend walking without crutches until patients can do so entirely normally. A normal gait means an observer should note neither limping nor awkwardness when the patient walks. This usually takes about a month after surgery. Perhaps even more important to the highway commuter, I also tell patients that when they can walk normally, they may drive again if the injured limb is on the right side.

Once patients decrease the swelling and gradually regain their range of motion in the knee, the goal of rehabilitation shifts to strengthening. The focus is closed chain strengthening (which means with the foot planted on the ground) and my preference is the leg press since it is safe and easy to do correctly. The patient starts off with low-impact activities like spinning on a stationary bike and later moves on to the elliptical machine. The strengthening program focuses on the quadriceps and hamstrings as well as the hip stabilizers and the core of the body. It is only when these muscles can adequately control the knee that patients should consider running. Patients who hit the treadmill too early often see their pain and swelling return.

Unfortunately, patients can't just push through it. "No pain, no gain" does not apply. Pain and swelling inhibit the function of the quadriceps, just another product of evolution that makes sense—if your leg joints are in pain, you probably shouldn't be running—but frustrates those who approach rehabilitation too aggressively. If the quadriceps are inhibited by pain and swelling, they atrophy and weaken. This reduces yet further their ability to stabilize the knee, leading to more pain and swelling during activity, which completes a vicious cycle.

If the patient makes sure to strengthen the quadriceps well enough before running, however, that cycle is avoided. This takes time, usually at least 3–4 months after surgery, and it is a gradual process. A rule of thumb I use to allow patients to return to running is the step down test, taught to me by our senior physical therapist John Cavanaugh at the Hospital for Special Surgery. I ask the patient to stand on a nine-inch (22.5-cm) step. I then ask them to lower their operated leg, heel first with their toes in the air. If they can repeat this exercise lowering the non-operated leg with the same amount of control, they are ready to start a running program. Patients start by running just a few minutes at a time, at speeds of no more than 5–6 miles per hour. Little by little, you crank up the speed, stay on a bit longer, and eventually begin to run every day. I hesitate to use exact figures or lay out a strict regimen, because patients progress at varying rates. If a run leaves the knee in pain and swollen, then you've gone too far and need to take some time off to recover.

Even without running, it is possible to get into trouble by going too hard, too early. A frustrated Sophia Taylor came to see me two months after reconstructive surgery, unable to figure out why she continued to experience pain and swelling even after working diligently to strengthen her leg muscles in physical therapy. A brief conversation revealed the culprit: her therapist had moved her onto the elliptical machine too early. Though it forces the knee to endure only a fraction of the impact which running does, elliptical exercise is still appreciably greater in impact than spinning. It is no substitute for the stationary bike. Six weeks back on the bike, followed by four on the elliptical, had Sophia running just over four months after surgery. The subtleties of rehabilitation are not to be overlooked.

Of course, running isn't all that athletes do, particularly the ones who have just had surgery and who plan to get back to the cutting and pivoting sports they adore. Even before patients run, they may engage in light agility exercises like shuffling, skipping, and jumping. As they begin to run and continue to build their strength, patients may ramp up the intensity of these agility drills until they transition to sports-specific exercises.

Developing in a gradual progression, these exercises are crucial not only physically but mentally, too. A basketball player, for example, would start off with individual drills like practicing her jump shot and dribbling in for a layup. When she's draining shots and driving toward the basket with the speed she enjoyed before the injury, it's time to call up a few teammates for some one-on-one or two-on-two half-court play. After getting comfortable at this scaled-down level—again, building up from an easygoing pace to full-on aggressive play—she can return to practice and, finally, competition.

Exercises like these, which involve the movements and thinking of the sport to which an athlete seeks to return, reawaken and develop the neuromuscular pathways that have lain dormant for months while away from athletics. But they also build confidence. After a break from her sport longer than she's ever had before, that basketball player will probably feel apprehensive about the game, unsure of her skill. This is something that patients completely overcome only with time and, really, only with competition, but the importance of the preceding sport-specific rehab activities cannot be underestimated.

The progression just described will be somewhat different for the patient who has had a meniscal repair in conjunction with ACL reconstruction. I will generally proceed a little more slowly with the initial rehabilitation, depending on the extent of the meniscal damage. While the ACL is fixed very solidly, the meniscus is merely held together with sutures that can retear more easily. In this situation, I will often limit weight bearing on the operated leg for two to three weeks and limit flexion (bending of the knee) to ninety degrees (a right angle) for four to six weeks, in order to give the meniscus a chance to heal without stress. After the initial few weeks, I allow the patient to rehabilitate normally, and, by four months, they are usually at the same level as those who have not had a meniscal repair.

BEGAN THIS CHAPTER BY NOTING the incredible variation among patients when it comes to their rehabilitation. Having then gone on to describe standard scenarios, I must return to an anecdote to illustrate the original point, which is an important one. More than anything else, good rehab takes attention by the individual patient. Sophia's case showed us that even a slight misstep in equipment choice can make all the difference in the world. In the following cases, not even shared DNA could dictate similar progress between two patients after ACL reconstruction.

Harry Klein plays football for his high school, and he plays it well. When you play football as well as Harry does, you don't want to miss one moment of a season; Harry sure didn't want to. So, he didn't. Harry was back on the field, leading his team as the star linebacker, no more than 5½ months after ACL reconstructive surgery. For most patients, this would be simply impossible. Return to sports takes at least 6 months on average, and, even then, patients are generally not in full competitive form.

Three things contributed to Harry's extraordinary recovery: attitude, work, and genetics. He was passionate about the activity from which his ACL injury had removed him so suddenly, and he wanted to get back to it, badly. More than that, the drive wasn't all in his head; he turned motivation into hard work, and put the time in necessary to strengthen his muscles to their former state. Indeed, it was hard work that had already brought him to a point of peak physical condition before the injury even occurred. But, there was one factor more important than either of these: what Harry was born with. Most seventeen-year-olds cannot achieve the musculature which he put to good use on the football field. Harry's legs could recover from trauma that much faster because they were just so strong.

None of these things was true of Harry's father, who tore his ACL two years after his son did. Bill Klein, an attorney from Connecticut, did not play an aggressive sport at a competitive level; he enjoyed paddle tennis as an important part of his social life. It was for this reason that he elected to undergo ACL reconstruction. Paddle tennis, though, was only something he did in the spare time he had between his office and the courthouse. Bill is part of a busy law practice, and his recovery coincided with a big trial. I mentioned earlier that, for adults, life can get in the way of rehabilitation; this was one of those times.

Bill had neither the passion for his sport that Harry did—it was a casual backdrop to social activity—nor the willingness to invest huge amounts of time in his rehabilitation—he had a trial to attend to! We cannot comment on Bill's genetics, as he shares part of them with Harry and may have been a veritable facsimile of his son at age seventeen. But, if that is the case, he had certainly gained by age fifty-one at least twenty pounds that he didn't need and lost at least that much of what he did need: muscle. Bill was not in great shape. Six months after his surgery, Bill was only starting to run on the treadmill. Fully one year had passed since his surgery before he was wielding a paddle on the court again. Different patients recover at different paces.

Bill's story also highlights an aspect of rehabilitation that contributes to its variability: the doctor's lack of control. In the operating room, looking through the scope and placing a guide wire for screw placement, the surgeon has a pretty good bead on things at the moment and can dictate what happens next. The patient sedated on the table certainly isn't putting up much of a fight. But once a patient leaves the hospital, all bets are off. Many patients find it difficult to find the time to complete their rehabilitation. Doctors who find themselves patients are the worst offenders, and I'm no exception.

It's only natural: if you feel like you can do something, you'll generally push your body to do it. In fact, it is the patients who categorically dismissed the advice of medical professionals thirty years ago whom we can thank for the more speedy recovery after ACL surgery today. What was originally referred to as "accelerated rehabilitation" is now the standard of care.[100,101] Sometimes, doctors are too conservative. In other cases, even patients can be overly conservative, afraid to damage the knee or experience pain.

Second only to doctors in ignoring doctors' orders are adolescents. Between twelve and fourteen years of age, patients are often in a precarious position of motivation without discipline. They really want to get better—many are already playing sports at a lofty level—but they lack the maturity to reign in the urge to push their bodies. Three months after ACL surgery, a twelve-year-old is not physically ready to play soccer again. But three months in the life of that twelve-year-old might as well be three millennia. They don't want to hear that three more millennia will come to pass before their cleats dig into dirt again. These young patients are liable to lean hard on their ACL grafts long before the tissue can handle it. Whether having picked up a basketball or hopped on a skateboard, some kids just can't resist getting back to their activities.

"What have you been doing on this knee?" I posed the question to thirteen-year-old Doug Fry, because I was perplexed; the graft was loose four months after surgery. The confusion only lasted until I recalled that Doug, while not a basketball player in any organized league, loved nothing more than all-out pick-up matches with his buddies. "Well, I've been playing a little on it, you know..." As a surgeon, that's not what you want to hear.

Doug's mother chided him, and the truth came out. Three months after he'd been sent home in a rigid brace, Doug had been playing aggressive full court basketball. And just over four months after that primary ACL reconstruction, he was back in the operating room. It's a free country, and patients can take liberties with their knees that they shouldn't. The best a surgeon can do is to ask them not to. Actually, the best a surgeon can do is to explain to the patient exactly *why* he can't take those liberties, addressing him as an adult. If the patient is not *actually* an adult, you do the same with the adults in the room: the parents.

If you think about it, the length of recovery time after ACL reconstructive surgery isn't even intuitive. After all, we're taking a fresh, live piece of tissue from the patient—if it's an autograft—and putting it right back in the body, screwing it in tightly, and closing everything up. Then we allow some time for the incisions to heal and the swelling to go down. But, if that ligament or tendon was working where it used to be, why won't it work in its new location?

The reason is purely biological, and biological processes are not always intuitive. At the very least, they require some elucidation before the subtleties become clear. What seems here to be a live piece of tissue isn't truly so from the moment we take it from its original location; to reach functionality, it must transform in a process called "ligamentization." It is true that, just after its removal, an autograft is quite strong. But, in severing it from its original blood supply, we effectively kill the tissue.

It is for this reason that something peculiar happens: the graft actually becomes weaker over the six weeks following its new placement, as its original tissue dies, and the cells in the new location have yet to populate it fully with new tissue. You wouldn't know it, because you can't see it happening, but the graft is actually just a scaffold which cells must fill with new tissue—and into which new blood vessels must develop—before it is truly functional. This process probably takes at least two years or more to complete fully, but we've found that the ligament is generally strong *enough* at about six months after surgery to consider return to sports.

Of course, some athletes can return at an earlier point, though cutting more than two months from that standard figure is extremely rare. Harry Klein, of whom I spoke earlier, certainly isn't the only example of a successful return less than six months post-surgery. Lana Kronman performed a similar feat after tearing her ACL in November of her junior year of high school. She wanted the same thing Harry did—to play her sport with her teammates when the season rolled around. In Lana's case, that sport was lacrosse, and the season was in the spring. That didn't leave a whole lot of time for rehab. Like Harry, she was motivated, hardworking, and blessed with a genetic endowment that simply made her muscles bigger and stronger than those of the average teenager. As Harry's story showed us, bigger, stronger muscles recover more quickly from the trauma of surgery. No more than 5½ months after walking out of the hospital on crutches, she was cradling the ball and whipping shots on goal. Lana was named Player of the Year that season. There will always be exceptions to the rule.

For professional athletes, there could be a great deal of money on the line—it could be worth the gamble. Most get away with that gamble. But, if they don't, the gamble certainly hasn't saved them any time. It's like doubling the speed limit to get to a wedding: if you're lucky, you'll get there a lot faster. If you're not, you'll be spending plenty of time—way more time than you saved by putting the pedal to the metal—in conversation with a state trooper.

Graft re-tear brings with it the possibility of another surgery and the certainty of many more months of rehabilitation. While the chances that it will happen are relatively low, those chances grow dramatically when athletes reduce their time in rehab to the bare minimum.

THE THREE MOST COMMON CAUSES of ACL graft re-injury are traumatic, biological, and technical. First, let's review the traumatic case. If you can tear your original ACL, you can certainly tear the reconstructed one. The same moves on the field or court that injure the normal tissue can tear the grafted tissue as well. Secondly, biology is the culprit in other cases, as the graft may not heal as well as we would like for many reasons. It makes sense that allograft (that is, transplanted tissue from a cadaver) heals more slowly, since it is not the patient's own. Rejection is generally not an issue for orthopedic tissues as it is for transplanted livers and kidneys, but there may be a small reaction from the patient's immune system in some cases. Incorporation is slower for allograft as compared to their own grafted tissue. As well, soft tissue grafts (such as hamstrings) may heal more slowly to bone than a patellar tendon graft which has bone at either end. The bone at each end of a patellar tendon graft can heal to the patient's own bone like fracture heals. Soft tissue grafts may therefore be at higher risk of stretching or tearing than the ones with bone to bone healing that were taken from the patient's own body. Lastly, surgical technique is responsible for re-injury in cases where the graft was not placed in the proper position, or if it was not fixed securely enough.

In many cases, it is easier to re-do a failed ACL reconstruction that was not placed in the ideal location, because, in those cases, the prior tunnels and screws are out of the way, and the surgeon can easily place the graft in the correct position. If the prior surgeon placed the original graft in the ideal location, it is more complicated to re-drill the tunnels, since screws or other devices may be in the way. I actually enjoy revision ACL reconstruction, since I find it challenging, and each case is different. I often have to remove hardware to place the graft where it needs to go. In other cases, there is too much bone loss and hardware from prior surgery to adequately create new tunnels and fix the graft. In such cases, I have to put bone graft (from the patient or a donor) into the old tunnels, let the bone reconstitute, and then return six months later, when the bones are good as new and I can put my tunnels where I need to. I try to avoid this, since multiple surgeries are suboptimal for the patient's life and their recovery, but it is sometimes necessary for a good result.

Sounds complicated? It certainly can be. The point is simple: rehabilitation, whether after surgery or to attempt to avoid it, is vital to recovery from ACL injury and not to be taken lightly. Cut it short, and the price you pay may be measured in time, pain, anxiety, and knee instability.

CHAPTER SIX

The ACL Prevention Program

YOU ONLY NEED TO WORRY ABOUT RECONSTRUCTING and rehabilitating an ACL if you injure it! All too aware of this simple fact, Dr. Grethe Myklebust and her colleagues at the Oslo Trauma Research Center set out to design the prevention program that is described in the chapters to come. I have been aware of ACL prevention programs for about ten years. However, like most of my colleagues, I didn't believe such a program could work. I thought that if you have an injury, the ligament will tear and exercises cannot possibly prevent the tear. I told patients that the programs were bogus if they asked. But all good doctors must have an open mind, and I now understand that the scientific evidence to support the effectiveness of ACL prevention is irrefutable.

I was first convinced of the effectiveness of prevention programs when I heard Dr. Myklebust's colleague Roald Bahr lecture at the 2008 ESSKA (European Society for Sports Traumatology, Knee Surgery and Arthroscopy) conference in Porto, Portugal. He presented their data that convinced me that their prevention program reduced the risk of ACL injury—without a doubt! The rates of ACL tears went down dramatically in the years when the program was implemented and it went up again in the years after it was stopped.

I met Dr. Myklebust less than two years after that conference. My friend and colleague Dr. Gideon Mann invited me to Jerusalem to lecture at his sports medicine conference that was held in January 2010. Dr. Myklebust was also lecturing at the same session so I took the opportunity to meet her and ask her about their program. Her understanding of ACL prevention is multi-layered in that she was a national-level handball player in Norway who tore her ACL and underwent ACL reconstruction on the injured knee. She is a practicing physical therapist and also takes care of the national female handball team in Norway. In addition to her personal and professional experience, she has carried out her research by personally instructing the athletes and their parents in how to do the exercises.

In my opinion, she is the world leader in this field on many levels. For these reasons, I asked Dr. Myklebust to become my partner in getting the word out about how and why ACL prevention programs must be implemented for our youth.

The program finds its roots in the 1990s, in Norway, and in a sport much more popular in that country than in the United States: handball. Dr. Myklebust understood then—as many more understand now—that ACL injury occurs by way of a specific mechanism, which I described earlier. That mechanism of injury would guide the development of the exercises to prevent its occurrence. Dr. Myklebust and her team set about determining the mechanism the best way they could, by asking numerous handball players to describe the movements they had made which led to their ACL tears.[102,103] It was this kind of research that eventually produced the information I related to you earlier in this book. A handball player would typically report that her ACL had been torn during one of two kinds of moves: planting one foot on the ground and exploding off of it in a cutting manner, or landing on one leg from a jump.

As I explained earlier, the mechanism itself—a characteristic forward shift of the tibia in relation to the femur—is identical regardless of the movement that causes it. For these purposes, however, it's just as useful to understand the more specific athletic motions that involve the mechanism, since these can be transformed into a program of exercises. Whether the game is handball or basketball, you wouldn't say to your athletes, "Hey, just lighten up on that anterior tibial translation during practice today." No, you would describe and demonstrate those exercises that would develop—both consciously and subconsciously—their ability to do just that. "Jump into the air, and try not to land knock-kneed." That sounds more like it.

Lest you think that handball players are the only ones who should be getting excited, notice that the athletic motions they described, while more specific than a general anatomic mechanism, are certainly not specific to their sport. You don't need me to tell you that cutting and landing from a jump are fundamental elements of a whole roster of other sports as well. If there's a wrong way to do either, which puts the ACL at great risk, there ought to be a right way to do either, as well. Figuring out the right way, then, and making sure athletes know it, could have broad implications; Dr. Myklebust and her team knew it.

Aware of the potential impact, and encouraged by the results of a study that had followed soccer players engaged in proprioceptive training—which increased each athlete's awareness of the relative position of her body parts—they moved forward with the design of their own prevention program.[104] The proprioceptive study exerted an influence, as it had been conducted with a similar goal in mind—to determine whether the program in question could reduce the risk of ACL tears. And if they aimed to influence the way athletes positioned their bodies in athletic motion—that is, teach them the "right way" I mentioned above—they would have to enhance those athletes' general proprioception.

Proprioception is most easily understood in terms of a more familiar concept: balance. Stripped of the ability to sense the position of one's own core and extremities all in relation to one another, balance simply wouldn't be possible without paying both conscious and constant attention to other indicators. Without proprioceptive capability, for example, it would be impossible to walk upright through a completely dark room, as there would be no visual indicators to compensate for the lack of internal indicators; balance would fail. That is, proprioceptive sense is entirely different from visual sense or any other of the oft-referenced "five senses," known as exteroceptive senses. Proprioception is a spatial sense modality completely internal to the body.

As any athlete knows, though she may not have been able to articulate it in these terms, proprioception can be developed with practice. The subtle, nuanced movements and controlling adjustments of any athletic action—which require conscious focus at first, but later become second nature—involve neuromuscular patterns that become effortless with repetition. The further these nuances and adjustments stray from a person's day-to-day physical movements, the more proprioceptive development they require. Furthermore, it is possible that, if pre-pubescent children are trained in proper and safe movement patterns, their neuromuscular pathways could be developed to protect them for a lifetime!

If we understand proprioception in the terms I described above, it makes sense that the study which sought to develop this sense made extensive use of "wobble-boards," or small platforms that are inherently unstable. Any action performed while standing atop a wobble-board requires the enhanced proprioception I just described, as the ground now moves! A principle conveyed so well by any of a thousand martial arts films, in which the fighter must practice his art not on level ground, but while standing atop a narrow column. Similarly, exercises atop the wobble-board develop proprioception, such that balance, control, and awareness suddenly become a whole lot easier when the ground *doesn't* wobble!

Of course, Dr. Myklebust did not forget what they had learned from the handball players themselves, valuable feedback that had been corroborated by video analysis.[37] Their prevention program would have to progress from general proprioceptive training to the athletic actions themselves: planting and cutting, and landing from a jump. Without a clear directive on how to apply enhanced proprioception to the movements of the sport, any wobble-board work would be far less useful. An athlete with merely the latter would be equipped similarly to the pilot whose aircraft can tell him his altitude to the nearest millimeter, but who hasn't the faintest notion of how high he should be flying!

For an ACL prevention program to be effective, the instructions must be simple. Especially when dealing with young athletes, it's a good idea not to let things get too complicated. Well aware of this, the Norwegian team developed a phrase that encompassed much of what the program sought to accomplish, and which eventually became something of a mantra: "Knee over toe."

If an athlete focuses on maintaining her knee in a position above her toe—rather than bowed away from it laterally (bowed legged position) or buckled inward from it medially (knock knee position)—the tibia is much less likely to slide forward of the femur to tear the ACL. It is particularly the knock-kneed, or valgus position that should be avoided; in fact, the Norwegian group let this particular tenet guide them before there existed the substantial evidence we have today that valgus leg geometry (that is the knock knee position), at least in the world of ACL injury, is public enemy number one.[105]

So, what did they come up with in the end to eliminate the knock knee (valgus) position, among other risky movements? Well, the program was finalized to include three kinds of exercises, each of which increased in difficulty through five stages; but the effects of the program on injury prevention were not easy to discern.[4] The general scheme made sense: exercises divided among wobble-boards, the floor, and balance mats as a transition between the two; each exercise carefully tailored to improve awareness and knee control during standing, cutting, jumping, and landing; and each group of exercises designed with progress in mind as the athletes developed their proprioception and strength. It seemed like it ought to work, but any evidence lacked statistical significance. The problem? Compliance. The same way medication won't work if the patient doesn't take it and surgery won't work if the patient doesn't follow the surgeon's post-operative instructions—the prevention program won't work if the athlete doesn't do it.

If athletes don't actually use a prevention program enough, it's hard to tell whether it works. Noting that some teams were skipping the prevention exercises but continuing with their regular warm-up exercises, the research group decided to recreate the program as a stand-alone warm-up program,[3] by including running exercises. This changed the program from a set of additional exercises to a part of the athlete's normal warm-up routine that is performed at every training session. It also turns out that young athletes get bored doing the same thing over and over again. I don't blame them. So, Dr. Myklebust and her team threw in more exercises to provide progression and allow coaches to shake things up. They also shifted the goal and reason for the program to focus on performance enhancement, rather than on injury prevention alone.

Did it work? In a word, yes. And we Americans will be happy to know that the later trial was conducted among players of a sport with which we're a bit more familiar: soccer. The study not only achieved 77% compliance—up from numbers as low as 26% in the first go-round—but found that female soccer players who participated in the prevention program were significantly less likely injure themselves, by more than a third, in fact.[3] An earlier study had already shown that acute knee or ankle injuries could be reduced by

50% and severe injuries by an even greater margin.[5] The numbers were, and still are, extremely impressive.

But let's not limit the discussion to the studies performed by Dr. Myklebust and her group; let's take a look at the broader body of data on the subject. Even more impressive than the Norwegians' numbers alone are those presented by Dr. Jay Hertel at the 2010 meeting of the American Orthopaedic Society for Sports Medicine.[15] Hertel analyzed seven studies of ACL-injury prevention programs that had been conducted between 1999 and 2008, selected for their quality and representing over 12,000 athletes. He found that, on average, participation in this kind of program reduced the risk of noncontact ACL injury by a staggering 71%.

ACL injuries are the focus of this book since, as the data show, a huge number of them can be prevented by the program. But the prevention program does not merely reduce the risk of major knee injuries. By focusing on core stability, balance, and neuromuscular control, it also cuts down on ankle and overuse injuries that keep athletes off the field just as often.[3] If I sound like a salesman, and you are waiting for the catch, I'm sorry to disappoint you: there is none. All it takes is the discipline to do the exercises, and your risk goes down. By a lot. It really is that simple. We have no more time to lose—it is time to implement these programs for all athletes at risk. In fact, why not have all kids do the exercises in their gym classes at school? Anything less would be downright irresponsible.

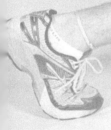

CHAPTER SEVEN

Strength, Balance, and Plyometrics

A ND NOW, THE GOOD STUFF.

At long last, here is the information to which I have alluded throughout the book so far: the ACL injury prevention exercises. While the program has been developed through a number of iterations, as I touched on in the last chapter, you will find here a version that draws on Dr. Myklebust's program but is modified to provide even more variation and progression, to keep athletes interested and engaged, something which is crucial to the success of any program like this one. In this chapter, I will list and describe the exercises that focus on balance, strength, and plyometrics.

That last term still needs explaining. Balance is crucial to sports injury prevention in general, as I explained earlier in relation to proprioceptive training. Strength carries an importance that is more intuitive (knowing where to place your knee in relation to your toes, and possessing the balance to realize what you know, is patently useless if your muscles are too weak to achieve that position). However, plyometric training is more subtle. It combines both neurological and muscular development for one purpose: speed. We've heard of *explosive* strength—plyometrics help to attain it. Plyometrics training is commonly used to improve athletic performance; it is an established technique for increasing vertical jump height and sprint speed, necessary for sports such as basketball. Luckily for us these exercises not only improve performance but also help to protect the ACL. Just as an athlete must have an *awareness* of her limbs' relative locations and the *strength* to re-orient her limbs into a safe position, she must be able to do so *quickly*, if she aims to avoid injury.

The exercises in this chapter cultivate these three elements of injury prevention. Each type of strengthening exercise progresses through three levels of intensity, and each type of balance and plyometric exercise, through five levels; I will describe them all. When you perform the program, you should pick the level that feels comfortable yet also presents a challenge. This level will vary based on your age and strength. As I mentioned in the last chapter, young athletes enjoy programs that are varied and progressive in this way.[3] Even when a child has a computer joystick in hand rather than a ball, she'll tell you that levels really push her to concentrate! Getting better is fun; quantifying the improvement is engaging.

STRENGTH

The Plank

Level 1: Both Legs

I'll start off with an exercise you might be familiar with, "the plank." The starting position is particularly important for this one, as the elbows must be placed directly beneath the shoulders to achieve the desired effect. If it's muddy out there on the field, you might get a little dirty. Lie on your stomach and place your forearms underneath you, hands on the ground with your elbows directly beneath your shoulders, as I stated before. That last part is the easiest to get wrong in performing what is, otherwise, a simple exercise. Once you have your arms properly located and your toes gripping the ground, lift up your entire body, supporting your weight on your forearms and toes. Make sure to pull in your navel, such that your body is in a straight line; you should neither arch nor sway your back. The hard part? Don't let go! Hold the position for a full twenty to thirty seconds, resisting the urge to let your belly sag or bring your elbows back.

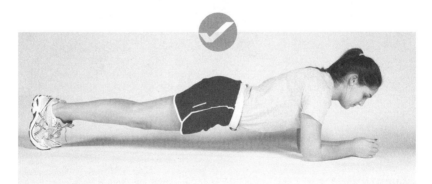

Photo by Nina Drapacz

FIGURE 1 Level 1: Both Legs—<u>correct</u> position with body held straight and elbows placed directly beneath the shoulders.

- Lie flat on your stomach with your forearms resting on the ground beneath you.
- Keeping your elbows directly underneath your shoulders, lift your body up so that your weight is supported entirely on your forearms and toes.
- Hold this position for 20–30 seconds.

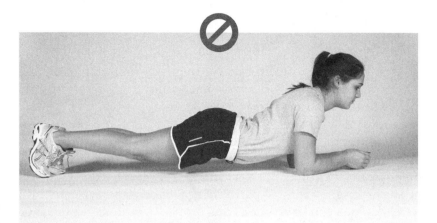

Photo by Nina Drapacz

FIGURE 2 Level 1: Both Legs—<u>incorrect</u> position with elbows placed behind, rather than beneath, the shoulders.

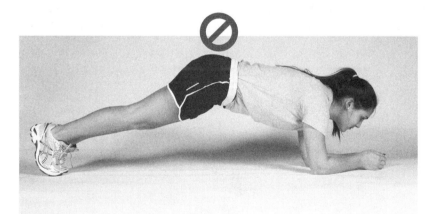

Photo by Nina Drapacz

FIGURE 3 Level 1: Both Legs—<u>incorrect</u> position with back arched.

Level 2: Alternate Legs

Again, take care to position your elbows directly beneath your shoulders before lifting yourself up, keeping your body in a straight line. This time, however, it is not just your trunk that gets a break from the dew-covered grass, but your toes, too! While continuing to make sure neither to arch nor sway your back, lift each leg away from the ground, alternating from left to right and holding each leg in the air for two seconds. You don't need to swing your leg high into the air; just hold each one a few centimeters from the ground. Be sure to also keep your hips aligned, and prevent your body from tilting to either side. Whereas in Level 1, your planted legs formed a straight line with your back, Level 2 requires that your lifted leg form a straight line with your back. Continue to do this for a total of forty to sixty seconds.

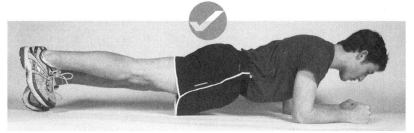

Photo by Nina Drapacz

FIGURE 4 Level 2: Alternate Legs—<u>correct</u> position with the lifted leg and back forming a straight line.

- Raise your body into plank position, supporting your weight on your forearms and toes, with your elbows placed directly beneath your shoulders.

- Lift your left leg a few centimeters off the ground. Hold it in the air for 2 seconds, and then lower.

- Repeat this lift for 40–60 seconds total, alternating between both legs.

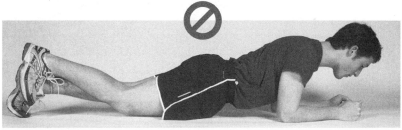

Photo by Nina Drapacz

FIGURE 5 Level 2: Alternate Legs—<u>incorrect</u> position with back swayed, held too low to the ground.

Level 3: One Leg Lift

This exercise requires you to pay attention not just to your elbow positioning and the straightness of your spine, but to your hips as well. Again, lift yourself onto your forearms and toes, maintaining the positioning details I described before. Then, as in Level 2, lift one leg away from the ground by a few centimeters. This time, however, you must hold that one leg in the air for a full twenty to thirty seconds, making sure not to let the opposite hip shift downward. As before, make sure neither to sway nor arch your back. After lowering one leg and taking a short break, repeat with the other leg.

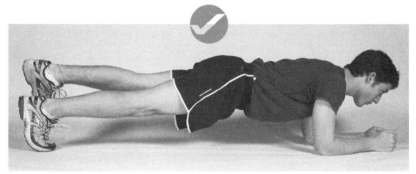

Photo by Nina Drapacz

FIGURE 6 Level 3: One Leg Lift—<u>correct</u> position with lifted leg held in a straight line with the back.

- Lift your body into the plank position as described before.
- Alternate between lifting each leg a few centimeters off the ground. This time hold the lifted leg in the air for 20–30 seconds before lowering and repeating on the other side.

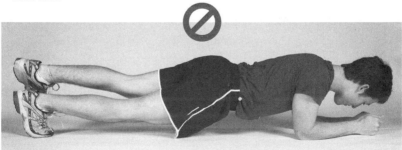

Photo by Nina Drapacz

FIGURE 7 Level 3: One Leg Lift—<u>incorrect</u> position with the hip opposite of the raised leg dipped down toward the ground.

Side Plank

Level 1: Static

This exercise is similar to the plank but, you guessed it, with your *side* facing the ground rather than your stomach. To start off, lie on your side while bending the knee that is touching the ground to ninety degrees, your lower leg pointing out behind you. When you raise your body, you will be supporting your weight on that knee and on your forearm, which should be resting on the ground, extending outward from your body. Here again, your elbow should be directly beneath your shoulder joint. Raise both your upper body and the leg that is not bent on the ground. That raised leg should form a straight line with the side of your body that is facing away from the ground, and the arm on the ground that you're using for support should form a ninety-degree angle with your upper body. In the end, your shoulder, hip, and knee on the lower side should all be in a straight line. I know, there are many angles involved, but you'll get the hang of it—just pay attention to where your joints are in relation to one another. Hold this position for 20–30 seconds, take a short break, and then repeat on your other side.

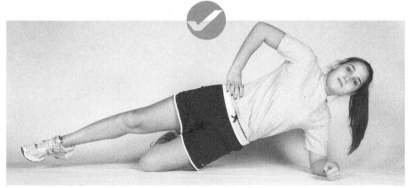

Photo by Nina Drapacz

FIGURE 8 Level 1: Static—<u>correct</u> position with lifted leg forming a straight line with the upper body.

- Raise your body into a side plank with your weight held on your left forearm and left knee. Your left leg should be bent with your left foot pointing out behind you.

- Keeping your right leg straight, raise it a couple of centimeters into the air and hold for 20–30 seconds.

- Turn over, now supporting your weight on your right forearm and right knee, and repeat the lift with your left leg.

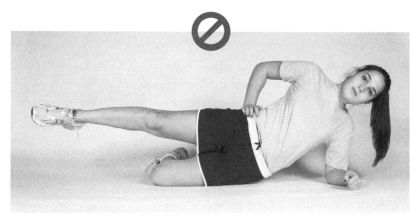

Photo by Nina Drapacz

FIGURE 9 Level 1: Static—<u>incorrect</u> position with hips dropped down toward the ground.

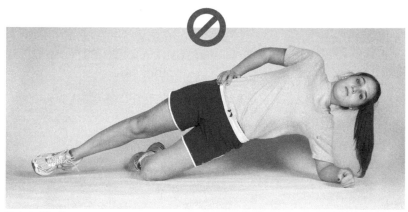

Photo by Nina Drapacz

FIGURE 10 Level 1: Static—<u>incorrect</u> position with hips held too high in the air.

Level 2: Dynamic

This time, keep both legs straight, so that you support your weight on your outstretched forearm—positioned at ninety degrees to your upper arm, with the elbow right beneath the shoulder—and the side of your foot. At the beginning of the exercise, your shoulder, hip, and foot should all be in a straight line. Instead of raising your other leg, as you did in the previous exercise, lower your hip to the ground, then raise it back up again to regain the straight line just described. Your other foot may rest on top of the foot that is supporting your weight. Repeat this dipping of your hip for twenty to thirty seconds, then, switch sides and repeat, with a short break in between.

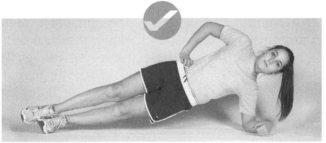

Photo by Nina Drapacz

FIGURE 11 Level 2: Dynamic—<u>correct</u> starting position with body held in a straight line.

- Beginning in the same side plank position as in Level 1, straighten both legs so that your weight is supported only on your lower forearm and foot.

- Lower your hips toward the ground, and then raise them to return your body to a straight line. Repeat this motion for 20–30 seconds.

- Switch sides and repeat.

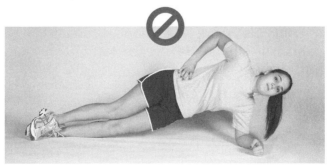

Photo by Nina Drapacz

FIGURE 12 Level 2: Dynamic—<u>incorrect</u> starting position with knees flexed, hanging toward the ground.

Level 3: With Leg Lift

Start off in the raised position in which you began Level 2, with your shoulder, hip, and foot all in a straight line. This exercise is similar to Level 1, except that you won't be using your knee for support. Again, the elbow of the arm that will be supporting your weight, should be directly beneath the same shoulder. Rather than dip your hip as in Level 2, raise your leg into the air, away from the one that is supporting your weight, and slowly return it to its resting position. Continue to raise and lower the leg in a smooth, controlled manner for twenty to thirty seconds. Take a break, turn over to your other side, and repeat the exercise.

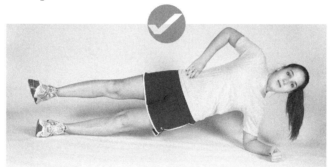

Photo by Nina Drapacz

FIGURE 13 Level 3: With Leg Lift—<u>correct</u> leg lift position.

- Return to the fully raised plank position as described in Level 2.
- Raise your upper leg into the air, and slowly return it to rest on top of your lower one. Repeat for 20–30 seconds.
- Turn onto your other side and repeat.

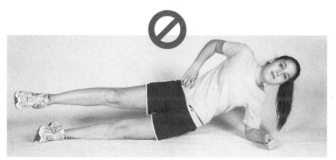

Photo by Nina Drapacz

FIGURE 14 Level 3: With Leg Lift—<u>incorrect</u> body position with lower hip dipped toward the ground.

Nordic Hamstrings

Level 1: Three to Five Repetitions and/or Sixty Seconds

This exercise takes two! Kneeling on a flat surface, whether soft ground or a mat, ask your partner to hold your ankles firmly. The most important part of the Nordic hamstring exercise is to keep your body perfectly straight, from your shoulders to your knees. Using the muscles in your buttocks and the back of your thighs to support yourself, slowly lean forward in a smooth, controlled manner. When you've leaned as far forward as you can, hold the position

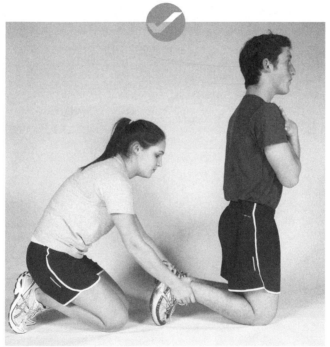

Photo by Nina Drapacz

FIGURE 15 Level 1: Nordic Hamstrings—<u>correct</u> starting position.

- Kneel on the ground with a partner holding down your ankles.

- Keeping your upper body straight, slowly lower yourself forward as far as you can. Remain there for as long as possible.

- When you can hold yourself up no longer, reach your hands down to the ground and gradually lower your body into a push-up position.

- Repeat 3–5 times, totaling about 60 seconds.

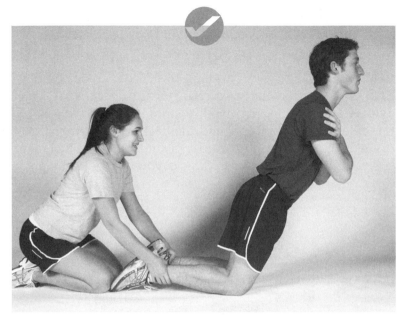

Photo by Nina Drapacz

FIGURE 16 Level 1: Nordic Hamstrings—<u>correct</u> midway position with straight upper body.

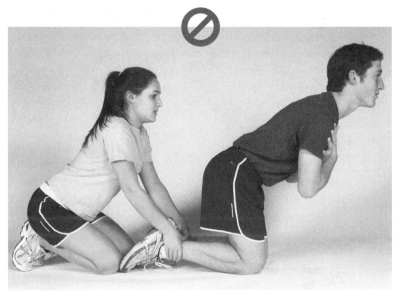

Photo by Nina Drapacz

FIGURE 17 Level 1: Nordic Hamstrings—<u>incorrect</u> midway position with hips bent.

for as long as possible. At the point when you can simply hold it no longer, reach out your hands and lower yourself down, gradually accepting your weight on your hands and ending in a push-up position. Complete at least three to five repetitions, totaling about sixty seconds in all. This exercise increases eccentric hamstring muscle strength, which is important as the hamstrings help the ACL during stopping and jumping. Building stronger hamstring muscles may therefore help prevent ACL injuries and decrease the rate of hamstring strain injuries.[106]

Level 2: Seven to Ten Repetitions

Level 2 is the same as Level 1, but requires more stamina. This time, complete at least seven to ten repetitions of the exercise. See Figures 15–17 for positioning.

Level 3: Twelve to Fifteen Repetitions

Level 3 takes yet more stamina! But the benefits are worth it. Complete twelve to fifteen repetitions, and feel the burn. See Figures 15–17 for positioning.

BALANCE

Now that you've strengthened key muscle groups in your core and lower body, it's time to work on balance. Balance training increases core stability and coordination. A well-developed core allows for better postural control, important for preventing both ACL and ankle injuries, and improves the transfer of forces throughout the body, which can improve athletic performance. In this series of exercises, you will also have to start paying more attention to your knees themselves, to avoid the at-risk positions that were described in previous chapters. Remember the mantra I quoted, "Knee over toe!" This will keep your knee flexed properly. Just as critical, do not let your knees cave inward! I will reiterate throughout the chapter this reminder to avoid the dangerous knock-kneed, or "valgus" position, but here's a phrase to keep in mind: "Never knock knees!" Repetition of these conscious and subconscious activities and reminders will eventually cultivate the good habits of movement that will preserve your ACL.

Single-Leg Balance

Level 1: Hold the Ball

Start off by standing on one leg, gripping a ball between your two hands outstretched in front. You can use a soccer ball, basketball, or whatever other kind of ball you feel most comfortable with. As you maintain your balance on one leg, rest your weight on the middle part of your foot, rather than on the ball or heel. Your supporting knee can be kept slightly flexed between 15–20 degrees. Crucially, however, do not let your knee cave inward! Remember the valgus, or knock-kneed position that was discussed earlier in the book? That is the position to avoid! Hold the proper position for thirty seconds, then switch legs and repeat on the other leg. Once you're confident that you can keep your knee in the safe conformation, you might get a little bit bored just standing on one leg. If that's the case, try passing the ball around your torso and underneath the knee that's not supporting weight, through your legs and back to where it was before, while maintaining your balance on one leg and concentrating on preventing your weight-bearing knee from caving inward.

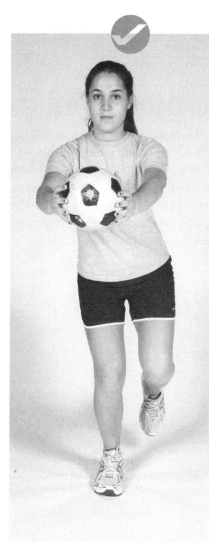

Photo by Nina Drapacz

FIGURE 18 Level 1: Hold the Ball—<u>correct</u> one-legged position.

- Stand on one leg while holding a ball outstretched in front.

- Rest your weight on the middle of your foot, flexing your knee slightly between 15–20 degrees.

- Hold for 30 seconds, and repeat on the other leg.

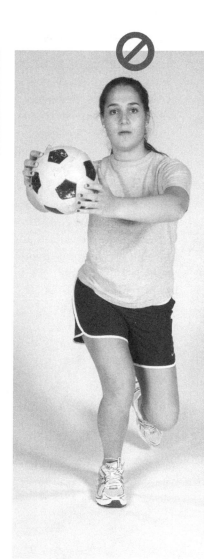

Photo by Nina Drapacz

FIGURE 19 Level 1: Hold the Ball—<u>incorrect</u> position with knees caved inward and hips dropped to one side.

97

Level 2: Throwing Ball with Partner

Isn't warming up more fun with a teammate? This exercise is particularly enjoyable not just for that reason, but because it more closely mimics the athletic movements you might perform in your sport. Stand about two to three yards from your partner, each of you balancing on one leg as described before. This time, however, pay particular attention to keeping your navel in, maintaining safe posture. Also, place your weight on the ball of your foot, rather than the middle part. Now, throw the ball to one another, remaining balanced on one foot and consciously keeping your knee from caving inward or extending over and beyond your toe. Remember, you want to avoid the risky knock-kneed position and keep your knee flexed enough to absorb shock. Think about these principles as you perform the exercise.

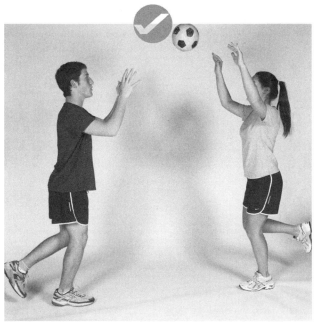

Photo by Nina Drapacz

FIGURE 20 Level 2: Throwing Ball with Partner—<u>correct</u> standing position with supporting knee over toes.

- Stand 2 to 3 yards from a partner, each balancing on one leg with your supporting knee slightly flexed.

- Throw a ball back and forth to one another while remaining balanced. Avoid the knock-kneed position.

Level 3: Test Your Partner

Isn't warming up even more fun when you get to challenge your teammates? While probably not as close to game-time behavior as Level 2—unless you like the sound of a referee's whistle—Level 3 is nonetheless a favorite, especially among younger athletes. Put the ball aside for now. Stand one arm's length from your partner, each of you balanced on one leg and keeping your weight on the ball of your foot. Now, while maintaining your own balance, try to push your partner off of her balance in various directions. You may push her on her shoulders, upper body or hips—any place that will cause her balance to waver. Again, keep your knee flexed and over your toe, and don't let it fall into the knock-kneed position! Continue to test your partner for thirty seconds, and then stop to allow both of you to switch legs. When you've challenged your partner on both legs, exchange roles and repeat the exercise.

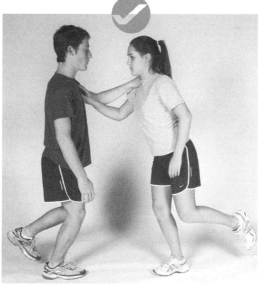

Photo by Nina Drapacz

FIGURE 21 Level 3: Test Your Partner—<u>correct</u> one-legged position while testing your partner's balance.

- Stand one arm's length from your partner, each of you balanced on one leg.
- Have your partner try to push you off balance in different directions. Keep your knee flexed. Do not let it cave inward.
- Switch roles with your partner and repeat.

Level 4: Throwing Ball with Partner on Wobble-Board

This exercise is just like Level 2, but with a twist—the ground will not feel solid beneath you! It's time to get out the wobble-board for an even greater challenge than before. You and your partner must stand atop the wobble-board, each on one leg, and throw the ball to each other as you did earlier. Take care not to lean sideways or allow your pelvis to drop on either side. Remember: "Knee over toe!" and "Never knock knees!"

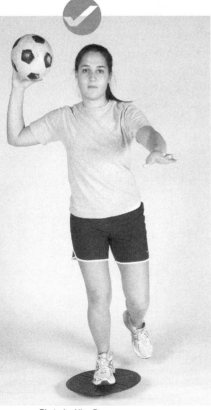
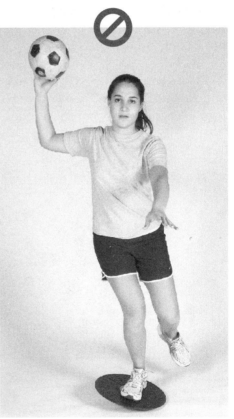

Photo by Nina Drapacz

Photo by Nina Drapacz

FIGURE 22 Level 4: Throwing Ball with Partner on Wobble-Board— correct knee position on wobble-board.

FIGURE 23 Level 4: Throwing Ball with Partner on Wobble-Board—incorrect knock-kneed stance with pelvis dropped to one side.

- Throw a ball back and forth with a partner while each of you stand on one leg on a wobble-board.

Level 5: Test Your Partner on the Wobble-Board

Just as Level 4 added the wobble-board to Level 2, Level 5 makes the balancing act of Level 3 even more difficult (and fun)! Both you and your partner step onto the wobble-board again, each standing on one leg, and attempt to push each other off balance. Be careful, as always, to mind your knees' positioning as described above.

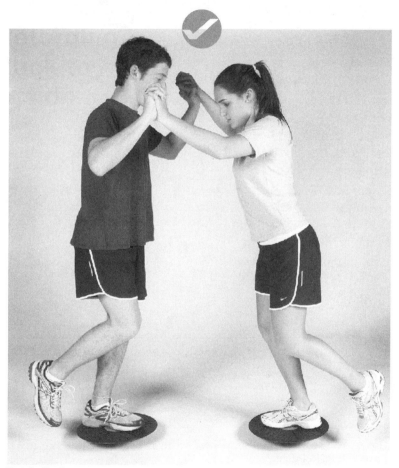

Photo by Nina Drapacz

FIGURE 24 Level 5: Test Your Partner on the Wobble-Board—<u>correct</u> position on wobble-board with supporting knee over toes.

- Attempt to push your partner off balance while you each stand on one leg on top of a wobble-board.
- Keep your supporting knee over your toes at all times.

101

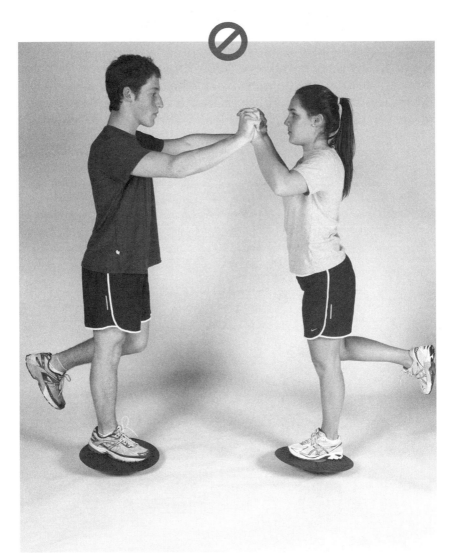

Photo by Nina Drapacz

FIGURE 25 Level 5: Test Your Partner on the Wobble-Board—<u>incorrect</u> position with supporting leg held straight.

SQUATS

Strength and balance are vital to injury prevention, but plyometric training provides the quickness of muscular contraction that can make all the difference in those fractions of a second that can mean either a close call or a tragic moment. The following exercises develop the explosive capability that every athlete needs. Levels 5 and 6 also include elements of the proprioceptive training on which the previous series focused.

Squats

Level 1: With Toe Raise

This exercise might remind you of sitting down in a chair, and that's exactly what you should imagine as you're performing it. Standing with your feet separated to hip-width, slowly bend both your hips and your knees to ninety degrees, being careful not to let your knees cave inward. Once in this position, straighten your hips and knees back out again, but more quickly. When you've completely straightened out your knees and hips, continue upward to stand up on your toes. Slowly lower yourself back down again to repeat the exercise. Continue for thirty seconds. Throughout the exercise, you may place your hands on your hips, if you like.

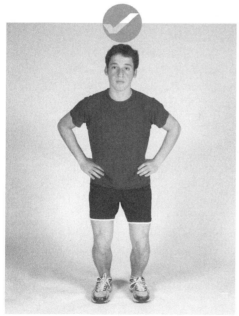

Photo by Nina Drapacz

FIGURE 26 Level 1: With Toe Raise—<u>correct</u> position bent at the hips and knees with knees over toes.

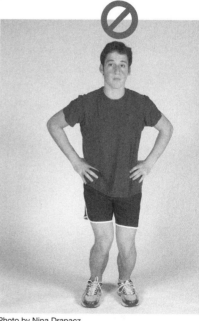

Photo by Nina Drapacz

FIGURE 27 Level 1: With Toe Raise—<u>incorrect</u> position with knees caved inward.

- Stand with your feet a hip-width apart. Slowly bend both your hips and knees to 90 degrees.

- Quickly straighten your body completely, continuing upward to stand on your toes.

- Repeat for 30 seconds.

105

Level 2: Walking Lunges

Here is an exercise you might be familiar with. Again keeping your feet at hip-width, lunge forward to the point where both the hip and knee of your leading leg are bent to ninety degrees. It is crucial to maintain both hip and knee control. Pay close attention—your knees should not cave inward at any point over the course of the lunging motion. Such valgus geometry can be easy to miss in this scenario, so concentration is necessary to avoid it. If you are practicing with a teammate or coach, have them evaluate your position. Make your way across the field in this manner, at a brisk pace, consciously stabilizing your hips and upper body to maintain a steady posture. Upon reaching the other side of the field, jog back to the starting point. If you're inside and near a mirror, you can also use it to monitor your movements at the beginning of this exercise, and then continue lunging across the room.

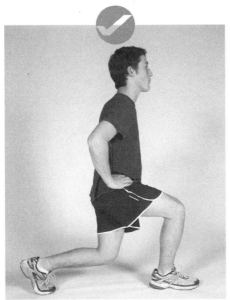 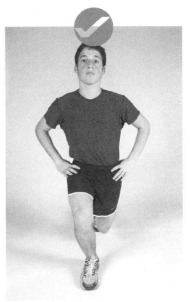

Photo by Nina Drapacz   Photo by Nina Drapacz

FIGURES 28 AND 29 Level 2: Walking Lunges—<u>correct</u> mid-lunge hip and knee position.

- With your feet separated a hip-width apart, lunge forward until your hips and knees are bent to 90 degrees.
- Continue to lunge your way across the room or field at a brisk pace.
- Jog back to your starting point when finished.

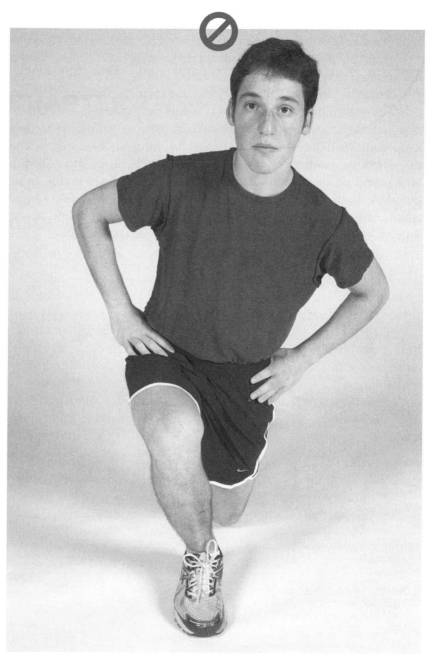

Photo by Nina Drapacz

FIGURE 30 Level 2: Walking Lunges—<u>incorrect</u> lunge position with hips uneven.

107

Level 3: One-Leg Squats

This exercise is simple but requires focus to be truly useful. While balancing on one leg, slowly bend your knee as much as you can, lowering yourself down in a careful, controlled fashion. At the point where you can bend your knee no further, extend your knee to raise yourself upward again, more quickly than you lowered yourself. You can do this exercise alone, or hold onto a chair, table or teammate to help keep yourself balanced. All the while, be mindful of your hips and upper body—neither should sag on either side. Even more important, pay close attention to the conformation of the knee that is doing the work. In this exercise especially, it is easy to let the knee bow outward or cave inward. Do your best to let neither happen! Bend down, and back up again, ten times. Then, change legs and repeat.

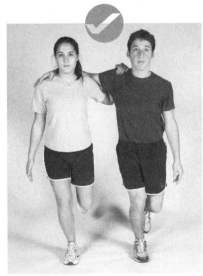

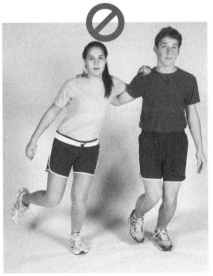

Photo by Nina Drapacz

Photo by Nina Drapacz

FIGURE 31 Level 3: One-Leg Squats— correct position with supporting knee over toes.

FIGURE 32 Level 3: One-Leg Squats— incorrect position with shoulders and pelvis uneven and knees caved inward.

- Standing on one leg, slowly bend your supporting knee as far as you can without losing your balance.

- In a faster motion, straighten your knee and raise yourself back to start. Keep your knee over your toes at all times.

- Repeat 10 times and switch legs.

Level 4: Squats with Toe Raise on Wobble-Board

This exercise builds on Level 1, destabilizing the surface on which you stand to add an element of proprioceptive training to what is otherwise plyometric. Remember, "Never knock knees!" Focus on avoidance of the valgus position as you lower and quickly raise your body. You can perform these squats for 10–15 seconds or, if you are able to, 20–30 seconds. Again, perform these exercises at the level that your age and strength allow. If you'd like to challenge yourself even further, close your eyes and perform these squats.

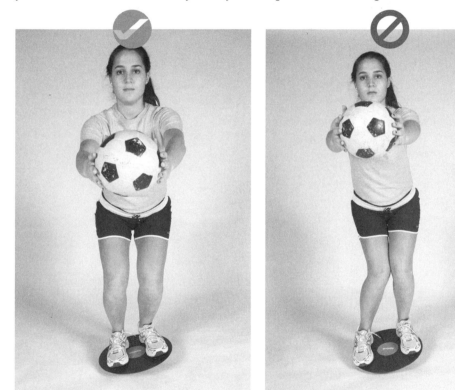

Photo by Nina Drapacz

Photo by Nina Drapacz

FIGURE 33 Level 4: Squats with Toe Raise on Wobble-Board—<u>correct</u> position squatting on wobble-board.

FIGURE 34 Level 4: Squats with Toe Raise on Wobble-Board— <u>incorrect</u> knock-kneed position.

- Squat while standing on both legs on top of the wobble-board.

- Quickly raise and lower your body for 10–15 or 20–30 seconds depending on your ability.

Level 5: One-Leg Squats on Wobble-Board

If you feel strong enough, instead of the squats in Level 4, try these one-leg squats. As a modification of Level 3, this exercise requires you to stand atop the wobble-board as you perform each squat using just one leg. Keep in mind the positioning guidelines as explained in Level 3! Be careful not to let your shoulders or hips become uneven or to let your knee fall into valgus. It is also important to note that these exercises can be performed without any special equipment. Instead of the wobble-board, stand on a balance beam or staircase

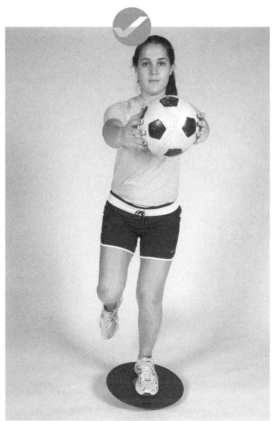

Photo by Nina Drapacz

FIGURE 35 Level 5: One-Leg Squats on Wobble-Board—<u>correct</u> supporting leg knee and hip position.

- Balance on one leg on the wobble-board.
- Perform squats for 10–15 or 20–30 seconds.

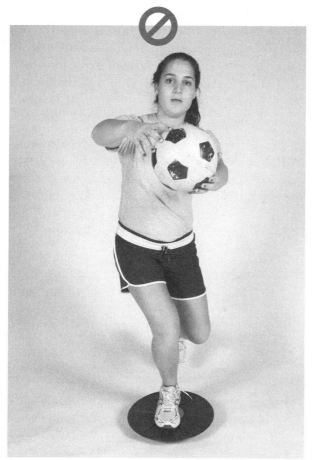

Photo by Nina Drapacz

FIGURE 36 Level 5: One-Leg Squats on Wobble-Board—
<u>incorrect</u> position with uneven shoulders and knocked-knees.

step so that one foot is parallel to the edge of the step and the other foot hangs off the side, hovering above the step below. You can also do it standing on a pillow. Perform the one-leg squats first on this leg and then turn your body 180 degrees to switch to the other leg. Or, to make it more challenging, rotate your foot so that it forms a ninety–degree angle with the step's edge and inch backward a bit so that only the front half of your foot is on the step. Your other foot should be hanging off the step behind your body. Now perform the one-leg squats for either 10–15 or 20–30 seconds, repeating with the other leg after you are done.

JUMPING

Level 1: Vertical Jumps

Think back to Level 1 squats, because this exercise requires you to imagine again that you are sitting down in a chair. Stand with your feet at hip-width, placing your hands on your hips if you prefer, and bend downward slowly until your hips and knees are at ninety degrees, just like you're doing a squat. Hold this position for two seconds, and use that time to check on your knees: are they caved inward? If the answer is, "No," then you're ready for the jump! Put your strength into it! Take to the air! Now, like any pilot will tell

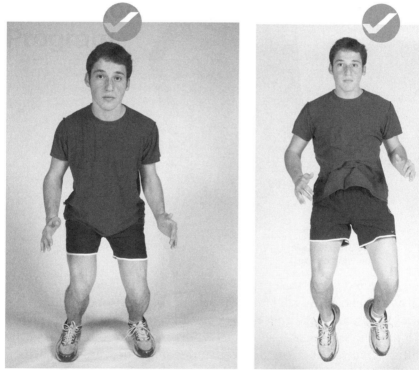

Photo by Nina Drapacz   Photo by Nina Drapacz

FIGURES 37 AND 38 Level 1: Vertical Jumps—<u>correct</u> landing and mid-air jump positions.

- Squat down until your hips and knees are bent to 90 degrees. Stay lowered for 2 seconds to make sure that your knees are not caved inward.
- Jump explosively into the air.
- Land gently on the balls of your feet with your hips and knees bent.
- Continue to squat and jump for 30 seconds.

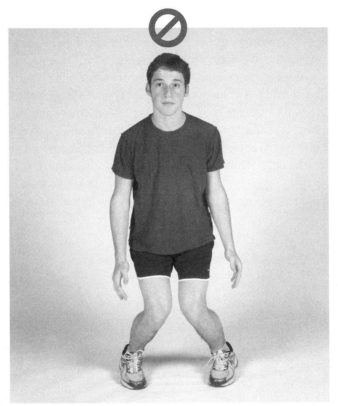

Photo by Nina Drapacz

FIGURE 39 Level 1: Vertical Jumps—<u>incorrect</u> knock-kneed landing position.

you, *landing* is the hard part. The goal is to land gently on the balls of your feet. In this "soft landing," make sure to bend your hips and knees, and take care to deliberately avoid the valgus position. "Never knock knees"—don't let your knees cave in towards the other. Continue to lower yourself and explode upward in this manner for thirty seconds. Remember that landing from a jump is one of the ways in which athletes typically tear their ACLs. This exercise will encourage you to land on two legs and increase your knee and hip flexion, which can reduce your chances of tearing your ACL. It deserves consistent focus and is one of the most important of the entire program. This is particularly true for young children because they can be taught how to land from a jump correctly at an early age, potentially setting their technique for life.

Level 2: Lateral Jumps

Cutting is another good way to tear your ACL, if you do it wrong, that is. This exercise mimics the lateral motion and sudden acceleration of cutting, and is designed to teach you how to do it in a way that will save your ACL. Stand on one leg with your hips and knees bent slightly, leaning your upper body marginally forward by bending at the waist. Jump sideways about a meter, landing on the ball of your other foot and coming to the position just described. Taking great care not to let either knee cave inward, as it flexes to cushion the landing and extends to push you back upward, continue to jump in this way for thirty seconds.

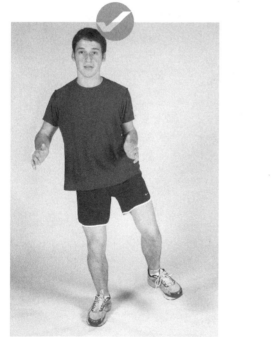
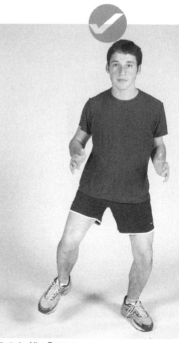

Photo by Nina Drapacz　　　　　　Photo by Nina Drapacz

FIGURES 40 AND 41 Level 2: Lateral Jumps—<u>correct</u> right and left leg landing positions.

- Bend your hips and knees slightly while standing on one leg.
- Push off of that leg to jump about a meter sideways.
- Land on the ball of your other foot with your hips and knees again slightly bent. Extend them to push yourself back up.
- Continue to jump from left to right for 30 seconds.

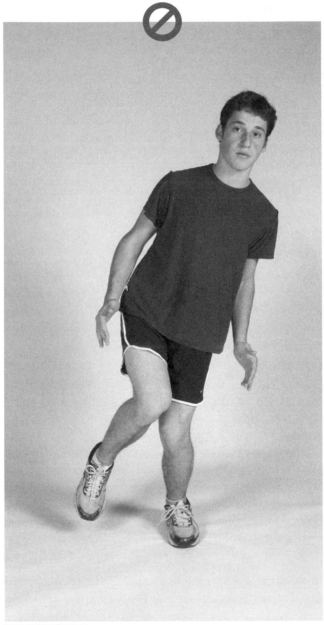

Photo by Nina Drapacz

FIGURE 42 Level 2: Lateral Jumps—<u>incorrect</u> knock-kneed landing position.

Level 3: Box Jumps

Imagine that you are standing at the center of a square painted on the ground. Use this mental image to help yourself cycle among three different kinds of jumping: from one edge of the square to the other (side-to-side), from the top of the square to the bottom of the square (front-to-back), and from one corner of the square to the opposite corner (along both diagonals). Continue to jump with your feet about hip-width apart, varying direction but completing an equal number of each type of jump, for forty-five seconds. If there is

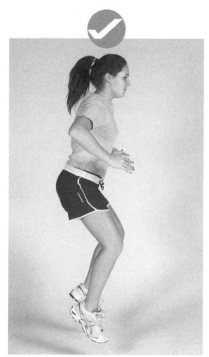
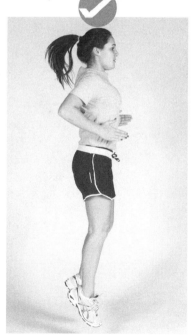

Photo by Nina Drapacz   Photo by Nina Drapacz

FIGURES 43 AND 44 Level 3: Box Jumps—<u>correct</u> mid-air jump position with feet hip-width apart and knees slightly bent.

- Picture yourself standing at the center of a square. Cycle among three kinds of jumps from one edge of the square to the other—side-to-side, front-to-back, and along both diagonals.

- Jump explosively into the air, landing on the balls of your feet with knees bent and over your toes.

- Continue to jump in varying directions for 45 seconds, performing an equal number of each type of jump.

one command that you should give to yourself as you perform this exercise, it's this: explode! Use all of the strength you have to jump as quickly as you can, erupting from the ground. Remember to land on the balls of your feet, and concentrate on your knees' geometry to avoid the knock-kneed position. This is plyometric training at its most obvious, the kind of exercise that builds explosive power.

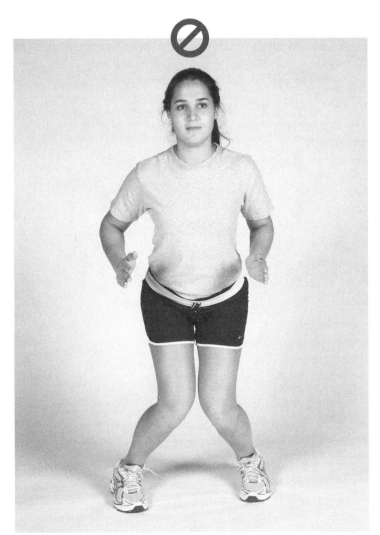

Photo by Nina Drapacz

FIGURE 45 Level 3: Box Jumps—<u>incorrect</u> knock-kneed landing position.

Level 4: One-Legged Jumping Sequence

This exercise combines agility with plyometrics. Jump forward on your right leg three times, then on your left leg three times. Finish by landing on both feet, taking care to bend both your hips and knees. Repeat this sequence five times to complete one set. Focus on quick, controlled, yet explosive jumps. And if the following is not in your head by now, it should be: "Knee over toe!" and "Never knock knees!"

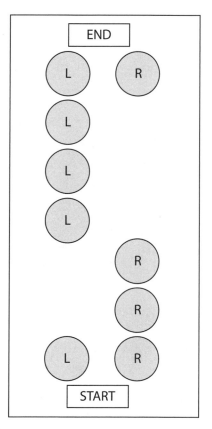

FIGURE 46 Level 4: One-Legged Jumping Sequence.

- Jump forward explosively on your right leg three times, then on your left leg three times.

- Bend at both your hips and knees with your knees positioned over your toes every time that you land.

- Finish by landing on both feet. Repeat the sequence five times.

121

Level 5: Box Jumps with Partner

If you enjoyed Level 3, and you love a good one-on-one challenge, then Level 5 will be right up your alley. As you continuously perform your front-to-back, side-to-side, and diagonal jumps, your partner will suddenly push you at the peak of your ascent in a direction that you cannot predict! Your partner should not push you every time you jump. This will make the push unexpected as well as unpredictable in direction. Your task is to land in a controlled manner that preserves your ACL: on the balls of both feet at the same time, hips and knees bent, and making sure not to let your knees cave inward.

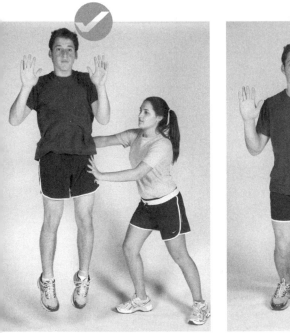

Photo by Nina Drapacz   Photo by Nina Drapacz

FIGURES 47 AND 48 Level 5: Box Jumps with Partner—<u>correct</u> mid-air jumping position with partner's push (on left) and <u>correct</u> landing position (on right).

- Continuously perform the front-to-back, side-to-side, and diagonal jumps as in Level 3.
- Have a partner suddenly push you at the height of your jump, varying the direction of her push.
- Land on the balls of both feet with your hips and knees bent, keeping your knees from caving inward.
- Continue for 45 seconds, and then switch roles with your partner and repeat.

Keep your knees over your toes and never knock knees! Cycle among the different types of jumps for at least forty-five seconds, then switch roles with your partner.

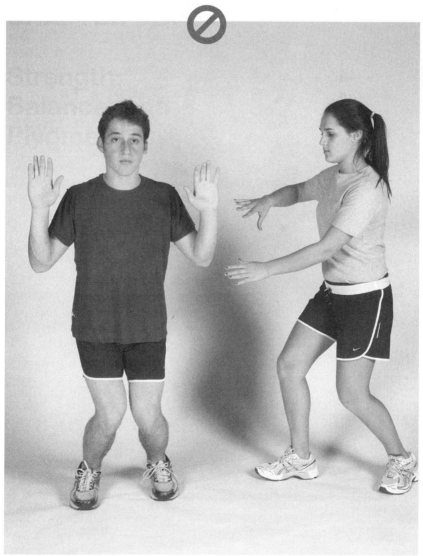

Photo by Nina Drapacz

FIGURE 49 Level 5: Box Jumps with Partner—<u>incorrect</u> landing position with knees caved inward.

CHAPTER EIGHT

Running Exercises and Program Scheme

REMEMBER THAT ATHLETIC PROGRAMS, and athletes themselves, are much more likely to comply with a prevention program when it can stand on its own as a comprehensive warm-up routine.[3] To that end, the program presented here includes a number of running exercises that also do their part to build strength where it is needed, improving athletic performance and imprinting in the neuromuscular pathways of young athletes the techniques to move and land that will preserve their ACLs for the long term.

RUNNING OVER FIELD

Bounding Run

This run goes like it sounds: take high, bounding steps, lifting each knee high into the air. Take care to land gently on the balls of your feet in order to reduce shock on your lower joints. At the same time, exaggerate the swing of the arm opposite the leg that is taking the leaping step. It is important to make sure that this leading leg does not cross the middle of your body; it should move upward and forward, not inward. Similarly, make sure that your knees do not cave inward as they endure these amplified motions. Keep knees over toes at all times. When you reach the other end of the field, jog back to recover.

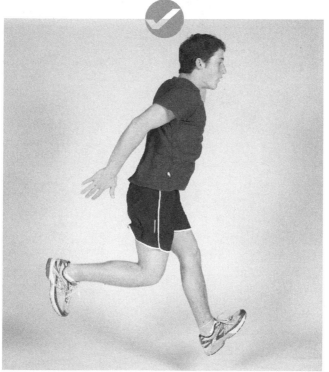

Photo by Nina Drapacz

FIGURE 50 Bounding Run—<u>correct</u> position in mid-air with legs not crossing the midline of the body.

- Take high, bounding steps as you run across the field, lifting each knee high into the air.

- Swing the arm opposite of your leading leg and land gently on the balls of your feet.

- Do not allow your legs to move sideways and cross the middle of your body or your knees to cave inward

Running and Cutting

This exercise is critical. Cutting movements when not performed properly can cause both harm to the knee and ankle sprain injuries. The lateral jumps described above help to cultivate good cutting habits, and it is here that those habits should be employed. Jog four to five steps, then plant one foot to make a hard cut, changing direction. Accelerate explosively in that direction, sprinting five to

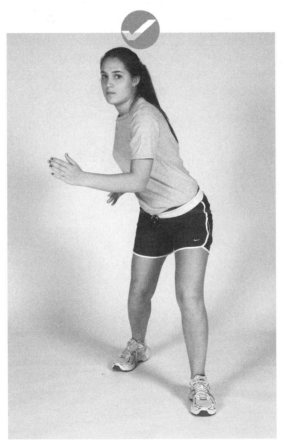

Photo by Nina Drapacz

FIGURE 51 Running and Cutting—<u>correct</u> cutting position with knees over toes.

- Jog 4 or 5 steps. Plant one foot to make a hard cut, changing direction.
- Accelerate explosively in the new direction, sprinting 5 to 7 steps before slowing down to plant the other foot and repeat in the opposite direction.
- Continue until you reach the other side of the field, and jog back to the start.

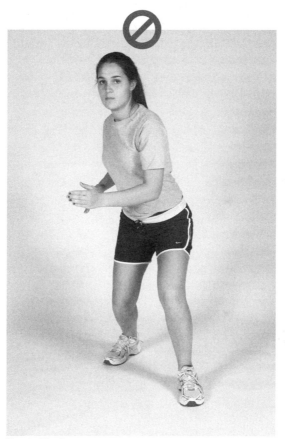

Photo by Nina Drapacz

FIGURE 52 Running and Cutting—<u>incorrect</u> position with the knee of the planted foot caving inward into valgus position.

seven steps at eighty to ninety percent pace before slowing down to repeat, planting the other foot to make another hard cut. Repeat this process until you reach the other side of the field, and jog back to the starting point. It is crucial that you focus on your knees' positioning throughout this exercise. Keep each knee over the toe beneath it, and avoid the knock-kneed stance! But don't forget the importance of your upper body. Remember to maintain a steady upper posture without allowing your upper half to sway too much to either side. Because cutting is precisely the activity that could end your athletic career, this exercise deserves your undivided attention. Repeat to yourself: "Knee over toe!" and "Never knock knees!"

RUNNING THROUGH COURSE

There running exercises require a set of six to ten pairs of cones, arranged in two parallel lines approximately five to six yards apart. Each exercise should be completed twice and can be performed in pairs, both players starting at the same time at the first pair of cones. As you warm up, you may increase the speed with which you cover the return part of the run to arrive back at that first pair.

Hip Out

Either walking or jogging at a nice and easy pace, stop between each pair of cones to lift your knee and rotate your hip outward. Alternate between your left and right leg. Done right, this exercise helps to build good pivoting habits and also provides a good warm up for sensitive hip muscles, useful for those who play sports like soccer.

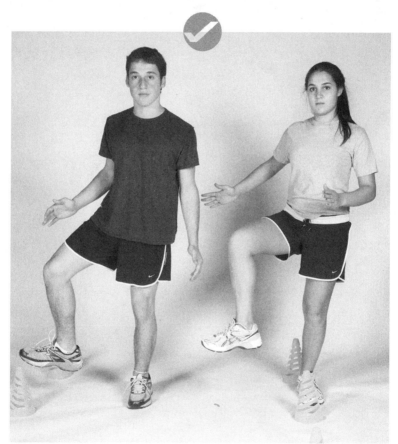

Photo by Nina Drapacz

FIGURE 53 Hip Out—correct position with knee lifted and hip rotated outward.

- Set up two parallel lines of 6 to 10 cones about 5 to 6 yards apart.
- While walking or jogging between the cones, lift your knee and rotate your hip outward between each pair of cones.
- Alternate between your left and right leg until you come to the end of the cones.

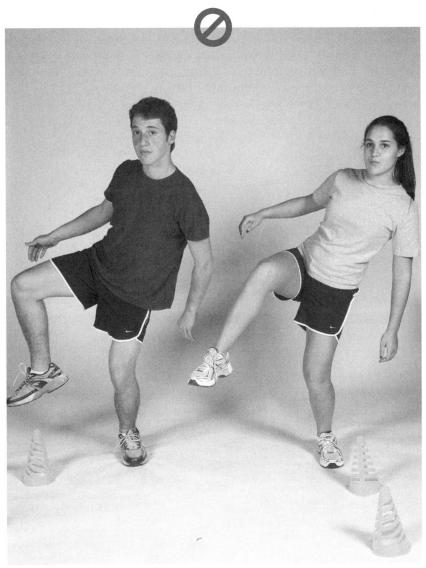

Photo by Nina Drapacz

FIGURE 54 Hip Out—<u>incorrect</u> position with supporting knee caved inward.

Hip In

This exercise is the same as the one just described, with one exception: once you've lifted your knee, rotate your hip *inward*. Again, alternate between your left and right leg.

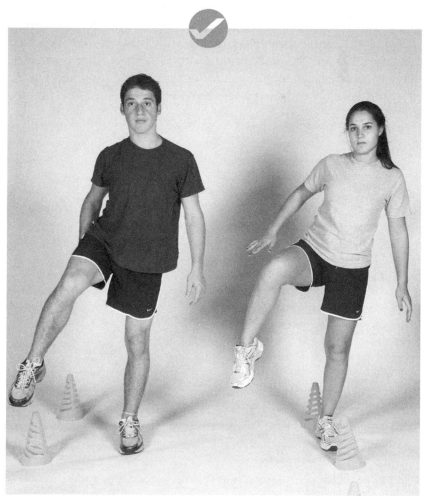

Photo by Nina Drapacz

FIGURE 55 Hip In—<u>correct</u> position with knee lifted and hip rotated inward.

- Perform the same knee lifts as in the previous exercise, except rotate your hip inward after you've lifted each knee.

- Alternate between your right and left leg as you move between the cones.

Circling

Do you enjoy square dancing? If so, you're in luck, because this exercise may remind you of that old pastime! Pick a partner, and run forward as a pair to the first set of cones. Then, shuffle sideways, meeting each other in the middle of the course. Continue to shuffle an entire circle around one another, returning back to the line of cones where you started. Run with your partner to the next pair of cones, and repeat. Keep going in this manner for the entire length of the course, concentrating on these important principles: stay on your toes, keep your center of gravity low, and bend at the hips and knees! Keep your knees over your toes, and don't let the knees knock!

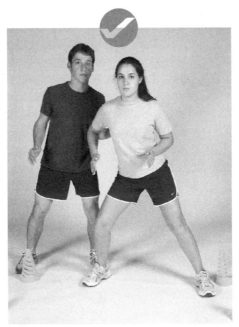

Photo by Nina Drapacz

FIGURE 56 Circling—<u>correct</u> position with knees over toes and bent at the hips and knees to keep your center of gravity low.

- Using the same cone setup as previously described, run with a partner toward the first set of cones.
- Shuffle sideways to meet each other in the middle of the course and continue to shuffle an entire circle around each other, returning to your original line of cones.
- Run as a pair to the next line of cones, and repeat.

Running and Jumping

This exercise starts off similarly to the last one—then, things get physical! Once you and your partner shuffle to meet each other in the middle of the course, jump sideways toward each other, making shoulder to shoulder contact in the air! As with the jumping exercises described earlier, pay particular attention to the way in which you land on the ground: land on both feet, and with your hips and knees bent, taking great care not to let your knees cave inward! You should make the jump a big one, and do your best to synchronize your timing with your partner's, such that you meet each other at the highest point you both reach and land at the same time!

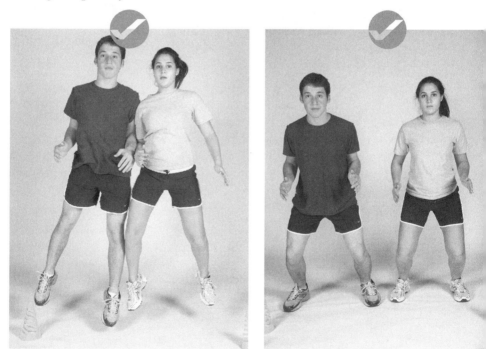

Photo by Nina Drapacz   Photo by Nina Drapacz

FIGURES 57 AND 58 Running and Jumping—<u>correct</u> position jumping into the air toward your partner (on left); <u>correct</u> position landing from jump with knees over toes and slightly flexed (on right).

- Shuffle sideways toward your partner and jump sideways to make shoulder-to-shoulder contact with your partner in the air.

- Land on both feet with your hips and knees bent.

- Synchronize the timing of your jumps with your partner's.

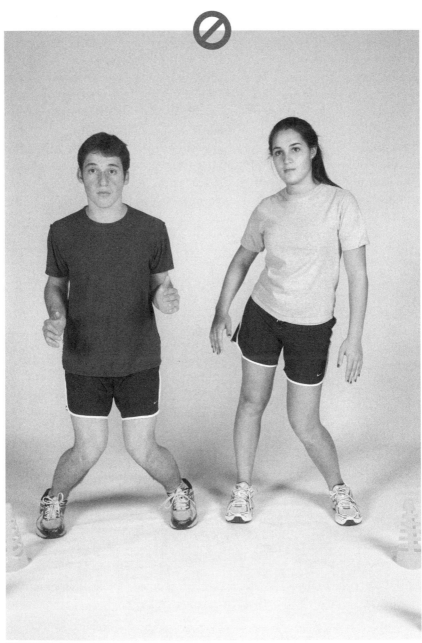

FIGURE 59 Running and Jumping—<u>incorrect</u> landing position with knees caving inward or knees straight.

Quick Run

The aptly named "quick run" is slightly more complex than it sounds. As a pair, run quickly past the first set of cones to the second set in the course. Just as quickly, run, facing backwards, to the set of cones just behind it, making sure to keep your hips and knees slightly bent. Continue in this manner—running two pairs forward and one pair back—until you reach the end of the course. Remember that your steps should be quick and small. "Knee over toes!" should be the phrase that guides you, and, as always, "Never knock knees!"

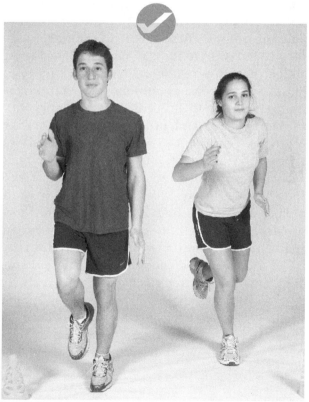

Photo by Nina Drapacz

FIGURE 60 Quick Run—<u>correct</u> running position with knees over toes.

- Run quickly with your partner past the first set of cones to the second set.
- Run, facing backwards, quickly to the set of cones just behind it.
- Continue to run forward and backward in this manner until you reach the end of the course.

ALL THAT I'VE PROVIDED SO FAR is a list of exercises, and you may be wondering how you should put them all together! Below you'll find the scheme of exercises that was found to be so effective when employed in the aforementioned 2008 randomized trial that was published by Dr. Myklebust and her team.[3] After players in this trial had become familiar with this scheme, it took about 20 minutes to complete.

It's important for athletes to incorporate strength and balance/coordination exercises into their training. I recommend that this exercise program be included in every athlete's warm-up routine. Adolescents who practice their sport 2–3 times a week should incorporate these exercises into each warm-up session and those who want to improve their balance and coordination should perform these exercises for 10–15 minutes, 2–3 times a week. But of course, coaches, athletes, and families should also adapt the program to fit their needs. **They can vary the exercises in the training sessions and progress from the easier to more challenging ones.** Feel free to recombine the exercises in a way that suits the sport, the athlete, the time available, or the practical circumstances. Some of the exercises in Levels 5 and 6 of the balance and plyometric sequences, for example, require balance boards or other accessories that you may wish to keep at home rather than bring to the field. **Use your imagination and invent other exercises that are similar to keep it fun. But remember to stay aware of the quality of your movements and positioning of your body when performing the exercises.** While the scheme that has been scientifically proven is always a good starting point, and this one is well suited to large-scale implementation, the most important objective is to be consistent in performing the exercises. And that's always easier when the program is tailored to individual needs.

COMPREHENSIVE WARM-UP EXERCISE PROGRAM[3]

Exercises	Repetitions
I. Running exercises, 8 minutes (opening warm up, in pairs: course consists of 6–10 pairs of parallel cones):	
Running, straight ahead	2
Running, hip out	2
Running, hip in	2
Running, circling	2
Running and jumping	2
Running, quick run	2
II. Strength, plyometrics, balance, 10 minutes (one of three exercise progression levels each training session):	
The plank:	
Level 1: both legs	3 x 20–30 seconds
Level 2: alternate legs	3 × 20–30 seconds
Level 3: one leg lift	3 × 20–30 seconds
Side plank:	
Level 1: static	3 × 20–30 seconds (each side)
Level 2: dynamic	3 × 20–30 seconds (each side)
Level 3: with leg lift	3 × 20–30 seconds (each side)

Exercises	Repetitions
Nordic hamstrings:	
Level 1	3–5
Level 2	7–10
Level 3	12–15
Single leg balance:	
Level 1: hold the ball	2 × 30 seconds (each leg)
Level 2: throwing ball with partner	2 × 30 seconds (each leg)
Level 3: test your partner	2 × 30 seconds (each leg)
Squats:	
Level 1: with toe raise	2 × 30 seconds
Level 2: walking lunges	2 × 30 seconds
Level 3: one leg squats	2 × 10 (each leg)
Jumping:	
Level 1: vertical jumps	2 × 30 seconds
Level 2: lateral jumps	2 × 30 seconds
Level 3: box jumps	2 × 30 seconds

III. Explosive running exercises, 2 minutes (final warm up)

Bounding run	2
Running and cutting	2

CHAPTER NINE

Frequently Asked Questions

If I am not doing the program, what can I do to prevent an ACL injury?

The basic principles of prevention include balance, strength, and position. These can be achieved with some simple exercises that you can even do while waiting for the bus or brushing your teeth. Start standing on one leg and hold it for a long as you can. If you are good at it, try with the knee that is in the air in a bent position. Try it with your eyes closed. Do single leg squats while watching TV. Hop around the room on one leg and make sure your hip is bent and that your knees are over your toes. Little kids can learn to jump off small heights and to bend their knees and keep their knees over their toes as they land. These are basic exercises that can develop good balance and good habits in kids at a young age. If kids are taught these habits very early on, these practices could persist into adolescence.

Can I train my child while she is young so that the benefits will last her a lifetime?

This question has not been scientifically studied. However, children learn motor patterns at a young age. If they are taught principles of ACL prevention (based on their age and maturity level) in gym class at their elementary and middle schools, it could well be that these motor patterns will forever be engrained in their brains and neuro-muscular pathways. In my opinion, these exercises can and should be implemented as part of gym classes for kids everywhere. There is no downside, and the upside could be enormous.

Can all ACL injuries be prevented with this program?

This program is mainly designed to prevent "non-contact" ACL injuries. That is, injuries that occur without contact by, for example, another player or an automobile. Non-contact injuries occur most commonly when planting hard to change directions or landing from a jump. The majority of ACL injuries that occur in sport are indeed non-contact, so this prevention program can have a profound impact. Studies have also shown that the total number of ACL injuries, both contact and non-contact, in athletes who do the program is reduced by half or more.

I tore my ACL. Do I need surgery?

For patients who have recently torn their ACL, the answer is "yes" if you plan to return to aggressive cutting and pivoting sports, such as soccer, basketball, or lacrosse. If you don't, but you are under twenty years of age, it is my opinion that people this age are active for so many years that they are very likely to develop instability, and you will probably be more satisfied following an ACL reconstruction. The same applies to people in their early twenties. As we get older, activity level tends to decrease. However, everyone is different, and there are some twenty-eight year olds who are completely sedentary and some fifty-eight year olds who are avid, competitive soccer players. For recent injuries, decision making is based largely on future activity level. If you have injured your knee and torn the ACL in the past and now can't trust the knee due to recurrent instability, surgery is a great option to eliminate the problem.

How do I choose the graft?

Graft choice is an area of controversy in ACL surgery. In my opinion, allograft or transplant tissue is a good option for revision or multi-ligament surgery. In general, I avoid allograft in high-risk patients (very young and active), since there is a higher rate of re-tear in this population with allograft.[74] Allograft can be a good option for primary surgery in lower demand patients, such as patients over forty years of age who are not participating in contact sports. Patellar tendon graft from the patient's own knee has the lowest rate of re-tear, in my opinion, and I recommend it for the high risk patients.[51,63,85] Hamstring tendons from the patient's own knee can be used in all patients, but are particularly useful for adolescents with open growth plates. I use iliotibial band from the patient's own knee for pre-pubescent patients, who are typically eleven years of age or younger, in order to avoid drilling tunnels across their growth plates.[89]

I have torn my ACL. Will I get arthritis?

No one knows for sure. What we do know is that the risk of arthritis goes up the minute the ACL tears, whether or not you have surgery. We also know that the biggest factor that contributes to the development of arthritis is meniscus loss.[28,107,108] Recurrent episodes of instability frequently lead to meniscal tears, so surgery is appropriate for patients who are at high risk of instability. Ultimately, like everything else, the chances of getting arthritis are also largely based on your genetics.

I had my ACL reconstructed. What is my risk of re-tearing it?

It depends on your activity level. In general, younger patients are more active in terms of cutting and pivoting sports, so their risk is much higher.[36] The more you play and the harder you play, the more risk. Females are at higher risk than males, so competitive teenage female athletes in sports such as soccer, volleyball, lacrosse, and basketball are at the highest risk of all. If the risk for all comers is generally believed to be five to ten percent, it could be twenty percent or more for the highest risk group, particularly if they are not following a proper prevention program. On the other hand, if you are over forty and don't participate in any cutting and pivoting sports but instead concentrate on sports like cycling, golf and weight training, your injury risk is probably under five percent, irrespective of graft choice.

My child is growing. Can she have ACL reconstruction?

The short answer is yes, and she probably should, pending other circumstances. Kids have a very high rate of meniscal tears and arthritis after untreated ACL tears. Certainly, any children who have recurrent giving way should have the operation. The problem is that kids often won't disclose their problem for fear of a trip to the operating room, and, if treated non-operatively for any reason, they must be observed closely by their parents for complaints related to the knee and signs of swelling, which can be telltale. Of course, the surgeon you choose to care for your child must be well versed in techniques that are safe for the growth plates, including "physeal sparing" and "trans-physeal" surgeries that put children at the lowest risk possible.

When is the best time to have surgery?

Ideally, you should have no swelling, or nearly none, and have a full range of motion. If you have surgery while the knee remains swollen and you lack motion, you risk developing a stiff knee, which can be a difficult problem to solve. This was often the case twenty and thirty years ago, before we realized the importance of restoring motion prior to surgery as well as the necessity of proper rehabilitation. It usually takes four to six weeks after the initial injury for the knee to be ready for surgery, but some patients can be safely operated on prior to that, and others take longer for motion to return. There are other factors which can force the surgeon to operate earlier, such as a displaced meniscal tear that must be repaired.

What if I stop doing the prevention program after doing it for a season and not getting injured?

Research shows that injury rates return to baseline if the athletes stop doing the prevention program. It must be done continuously. The most logical and efficient way to achieve this is to incorporate the program into the athletes' warm-up for practices. This way, they don't require the discipline to remember to do it, and they don't have to find a dedicated partner with whom to do it.

How long is recovery after surgery?

Typically, crutches are required for four weeks, at which point most people can walk normally. Strengthening is then required until the patient is strong enough to run, which is typically at three to five months after surgery. Return to sports is at six to twelve months.

There is significant individual variation, and there is a wide range from person to person.

Does ACL surgery hurt?

With modern anesthesia, the surgery itself is painless. There is discomfort for the first week or two that is treated with pain medication. After that point, most patients are relatively free of pain, although some remaining discomfort and stiffness can persist a little longer. Pain is also highly variable from person to person.

Will I return to my sport after ACL reconstruction?

Fortunately, the vast majority of patients are able to return to their sport after recovering from the surgery.

What sports are high risk?

There is some data available to support the following list,[109-113] but it is more of a general guide than a definitive rule. Risk is also related to the intensity and frequency of play and practices.

HIGH RISK (most common sports for ACL injury): basketball, soccer, lacrosse, rugby, American football, handball, field hockey, skiing, volleyball, squash.

RELATIVELY LOWER RISK (possible to tear the ACL, but not common): ice hockey, tennis, baseball, cross-country running.

VERY LOW RISK (almost impossible to tear the ACL in these sports): swimming, golf, cycling, jogging, weight training.

What can we do to prevent ACL tears in the future?

We can't prevent all ACL injuries, but we certainly can reduce the risk. Prevention programs should be implemented by all schools as part of their physical education curriculum. Kids in elementary school can do strengthening and simple balance exercises and progress to more challenging movements in middle and high school.

Kids' teams for high-risk sports such as soccer, basketball and others should implement the prevention program as part of their warm-up—so everyone does the program regularly. We have sufficient evidence to support the fact that this program reduces the risk of many different injuries in sport, particularly the devastating ACL tear. It is time to do it!

REFERENCES

1. Hewett TE, Shultz SJ, Griffin LY. *Understanding and Preventing Noncontact ACL Injuries*. Champaign, IL: Human Kinetics Publishers; 2007.

2. Shelton WR, Fagan BC. Autografts commonly used in anterior cruciate ligament reconstruction. *J Am Acad Orthop Surg*. 2011;19(5):259-264.

3. Soligard T, Myklebust G, Steffen K, et al. Comprehensive warm-up programme to prevent injuries in young female footballers: cluster randomised controlled trial. *BMJ*. 2008;337:a2469.

4. Myklebust G, Engebretsen L, Braekken IH, Skjolberg A, Olsen OE, Bahr R. Prevention of anterior cruciate ligament injuries in female team handball players: a prospective intervention study over three seasons. *Clin J Sport Med*. 2003;13(2):71-78.

5. Olsen OE, Myklebust G, Engebretsen L, Holme I, Bahr R. Exercises to prevent lower limb injuries in youth sports: cluster randomised controlled trial. *BMJ*. 2005;330(7489):449.

6. Soligard T, Nilstad A, Steffen K, et al. Compliance with a comprehensive warm-up programme to prevent injuries in youth football. *Br J Sports Med*. 2010;44(11):787-793.

7. Myklebust G, Steffen K. Prevention of ACL injuries: how, when and who? *Knee Surg Sports Traumatol Arthrosc*. 2009;17(8):857-858.

8. Brophy RH, Silvers HJ, Mandelbaum BR. Anterior cruciate ligament injuries: etiology and prevention. *Sports Med Arthrosc*. 2010;18(1):2-11.

9. Gilchrist J, Mandelbaum BR, Melancon H, et al. A randomized controlled trial to prevent noncontact anterior cruciate ligament injury in female collegiate soccer players. *Am J Sports Med*. 2008;36(8):1476-1483.

10. Silvers HJ, Mandelbaum BR. Prevention of anterior cruciate ligament injury in the female athlete. *Br J Sports Med.* 2007; 41 Suppl 1:i52-9.

11. Myer GD, Brent JL, Ford KR, Hewett TE. Real-time assessment and neuromuscular training feedback techniques to prevent ACL injury in female athletes. *Strength Cond J.* 2011;33(3):21-35.

12. Hewett TE, Ford KR, Myer GD. Anterior cruciate ligament injuries in female athletes: Part 2, a meta-analysis of neuromuscular interventions aimed at injury prevention. *Am J Sports Med.* 2006;34(3):490-498.

13. Myer GD, Ford KR, Hewett TE. Rationale and Clinical Techniques for Anterior Cruciate Ligament Injury Prevention Among Female Athletes. *J Athl Train.* 2004;39(4):352-364.

14. Myer GD, Ford KR, Hewett TE. Methodological approaches and rationale for training to prevent anterior cruciate ligament injuries in female athletes. *Scand J Med Sci Sports.* 2004;14(5):275-285.

15. Kronemyer B. ACL-injury prevention programs found to be effective for female athletes. *Orthopedics Today.* January 2011. Available from: http://www.orthosupersite.com/view.aspx?rid=79124.

16. Marx RG, Ryu JH. Displacement of the posterior horn of the lateral meniscus into posterolateral compartment: an unusual injury pattern. *HSS J.* 2009;5(1):9-11.

17. Bere T, Florenes TW, Krosshaug T, et al. Mechanisms of anterior cruciate ligament injury in World Cup alpine skiing: a systematic video analysis of 20 cases. *Am J Sports Med.* 2011;39(7):1421-1429.

18. Jarvinen M, Natri A, Laurila S, Kannus P. Mechanisms of anterior cruciate ligament ruptures in skiing. *Knee Surg Sports Traumatol Arthrosc.* 1994;2(4):224-228.

19. Krosshaug T, Nakamae A, Boden BP, et al. Mechanisms of anterior cruciate ligament injury in basketball: video analysis of 39 cases. *Am J Sports Med.* 2007;35(3):359-367.

20. Schechinger SJ, Levy BA, Dajani KA, Shah JP, Herrera DA, Marx RG. Achilles tendon allograft reconstruction of the fibular collateral ligament and posterolateral corner. *Arthroscopy.* 2009;25(3):232-242.

21. Stannard JP, Brown SL, Robinson JT, McGwin G,Jr, Volgas DA. Reconstruction of the posterolateral corner of the knee. *Arthroscopy.* 2005;21(9):1051-1059.

22. Stannard JP, Brown SL, Farris RC, McGwin G,Jr, Volgas DA. The posterolateral corner of the knee: repair versus reconstruction. *Am J Sports Med.* 2005;33(6):881-888.

23. Levy BA, Dajani KA, Morgan JA, Shah JP, Dahm DL, Stuart MJ. Repair versus reconstruction of the fibular collateral ligament and posterolateral corner in the multiligament-injured knee. *Am J Sports Med.* 2010;38(4):804-809.

24. Fairbank TJ. Knee joint changes after meniscectomy. *J Bone Joint Surg Br.* 1948;30B(4):664-670.

25. Hunter DJ, Zhang YQ, Niu JB, et al. The association of meniscal pathologic changes with cartilage loss in symptomatic knee osteoarthritis. *Arthritis Rheum.* 2006;54(3):795-801.

26. Tengrootenhuysen M, Meermans G, Pittoors K, van Riet R, Victor J. Long-term outcome after meniscal repair. *Knee Surg Sports Traumatol Arthrosc.* 2011;19(2):236-241.

27. Oiestad BE, Engebretsen L, Storheim K, Risberg MA. Knee osteoarthritis after anterior cruciate ligament injury: a systematic review. *Am J Sports Med.* 2009;37(7):1434-1443.

28. Oiestad BE, Holm I, Aune AK, et al. Knee function and prevalence of knee osteoarthritis after anterior cruciate ligament reconstruction: a prospective study with 10 to 15 years of follow-up. *Am J Sports Med.* 2010;38(11):2201-2210.

29. Arendt E, Dick R. Knee injury patterns among men and women in collegiate basketball and soccer. NCAA data and review of literature. *Am J Sports Med.* 1995;23(6):694-701.

30. Bjordal JM, Arnly F, Hannestad B, Strand T. Epidemiology of anterior cruciate ligament injuries in soccer. *Am J Sports Med.* 1997;25(3):341-345.

31. Ferretti A, Papandrea P, Conteduca F, Mariani PP. Knee ligament injuries in volleyball players. *Am J Sports Med.* 1992;20(2):203-207.

32. Gwinn DE, Wilckens JH, McDevitt ER, Ross G, Kao TC. The relative incidence of anterior cruciate ligament injury in men and women at the United States Naval Academy. *Am J Sports Med.* 2000;28(1):98-102.

33. Lindenfeld TN, Schmitt DJ, Hendy MP, Mangine RE, Noyes FR. Incidence of injury in indoor soccer. *Am J Sports Med.* 1994; 22(3):364-371.

34. Messina DF, Farney WC, DeLee JC. The incidence of injury in Texas high school basketball. A prospective study among male and female athletes. *Am J Sports Med.* 1999;27(3):294-299.

35. Dunn WR, Spindler KP, Amendola A, et al. Which preoperative factors, including bone bruise, are associated with knee pain/symptoms at index anterior cruciate ligament reconstruction (ACLR)? A Multicenter Orthopaedic Outcomes Network (MOON) ACLR Cohort Study. *Am J Sports Med.* 2010;38(9):1778-1787.

36. Lyman S, Koulouvaris P, Sherman S, Do H, Mandl LA, Marx RG. Epidemiology of anterior cruciate ligament reconstruction: trends, readmissions, and subsequent knee surgery. *J Bone Joint Surg Am.* 2009;91(10):2321-2328.

37. Olsen OE, Myklebust G, Engebretsen L, Bahr R. Injury mechanisms for anterior cruciate ligament injuries in team handball: a systematic video analysis. *Am J Sports Med.* 2004;32(4):1002-1012.

38. Wojtys EM, Huston LJ, Boynton MD, Spindler KP, Lindenfeld TN. The effect of the menstrual cycle on anterior cruciate ligament injuries in women as determined by hormone levels. *Am J Sports Med.* 2002;30(2):182-188.

39. Hewett TE, Zazulak BT, Myer GD. Effects of the menstrual cycle on anterior cruciate ligament injury risk: a systematic review. *Am J Sports Med.* 2007;35(4):659-668.

40. Hewett TE, Stroupe AL, Nance TA, Noyes FR. Plyometric training in female athletes. Decreased impact forces and increased hamstring torques. *Am J Sports Med.* 1996;24(6):765-773.

41. Lephart SM, Ferris CM, Riemann BL, Myers JB, Fu FH. Gender differences in strength and lower extremity kinematics during landing. *Clin Orthop Relat Res.* 2002;(401):162-169.

42. Wright RW, Dunn WR, Amendola A, et al. Risk of tearing the intact anterior cruciate ligament in the contralateral knee and rupturing the anterior cruciate ligament graft during the first 2 years after anterior cruciate ligament reconstruction: a prospective MOON cohort study. *Am J Sports Med.* 2007;35(7):1131-1134.

43. Flynn RK, Pedersen CL, Birmingham TB, Kirkley A, Jackowski D, Fowler PJ. The familial predisposition toward tearing the anterior cruciate ligament: a case control study. *Am J Sports Med.* 2005;33(1):23-28.

44. Griffin LY, Agel J, Albohm MJ, et al. Noncontact anterior cruciate ligament injuries: risk factors and prevention strategies. *J Am Acad Orthop Surg.* 2000;8(3):141-150.

45. Piasecki DP, Spindler KP, Warren TA, Andrish JT, Parker RD. Intraarticular injuries associated with anterior cruciate ligament tear: findings at ligament reconstruction in high school and recreational athletes. An analysis of sex-based differences. *Am J Sports Med.* 2003;31(4):601-605.

46. Daniel DM, Stone ML, Sachs R, Malcom L. Instrumented measurement of anterior knee laxity in patients with acute anterior cruciate ligament disruption. *Am J Sports Med.* 1985;13(6):401-407.

47. Potter HG, Linklater JM, Allen AA, Hannafin JA, Haas SB. Magnetic resonance imaging of articular cartilage in the knee. An evaluation with use of fast-spin-echo imaging. *J Bone Joint Surg Am.* 1998;80(9):1276-1284.

48. Buckley SL, Barrack RL, Alexander AH. The natural history of conservatively treated partial anterior cruciate ligament tears. *Am J Sports Med.* 1989;17(2):221-225.

49. Frobell RB, Roos EM, Roos HP, Ranstam J, Lohmander LS. A randomized trial of treatment for acute anterior cruciate ligament tears. *N Engl J Med*. 2010;363(4):331-342.

50. Levy BA. Is early reconstruction necessary for all anterior cruciate ligament tears? *N Engl J Med*. 2010;363(4):386-388.

51. Kocher MS, Saxon HS, Hovis WD, Hawkins RJ. Management and complications of anterior cruciate ligament injuries in skeletally immature patients: survey of the Herodicus Society and The ACL Study Group. *J Pediatr Orthop*. 2002;22(4):452-457.

52. Wester W, Canale ST, Dutkowsky JP, Warner WC, Beaty JH. Prediction of angular deformity and leg-length discrepancy after anterior cruciate ligament reconstruction in skeletally immature patients. *J Pediatr Orthop*. 1994;14(4):516-521.

53. Andrish JT, Cahill BR, Micheli LJ, Paulos LE. Extraarticular Reconstruction in the Skeletally Immature Knee. In: Pearl AJ, Bergfeld JA, eds. *Extraarticular Reconstruction in the Anterior Cruciate Ligament Deficient Knee*. Champaign, IL: Human Kinetics Publishers; 1992:24-34.

54. Aichroth PM, Patel DV, Zorrilla P. The natural history and treatment of rupture of the anterior cruciate ligament in children and adolescents. A prospective review. *J Bone Joint Surg Br*. 2002;84(1):38-41.

55. Mizuta H, Kubota K, Shiraishi M, Otsuka Y, Nagamoto N, Takagi K. The conservative treatment of complete tears of the anterior cruciate ligament in skeletally immature patients. *J Bone Joint Surg Br*. 1995;77(6):890-894.

56. Millett PJ, Willis AA, Warren RF. Associated injuries in pediatric and adolescent anterior cruciate ligament tears: does a delay in treatment increase the risk of meniscal tear? *Arthroscopy*. 2002;18(9):955-959.

57. Tayton E, Verma R, Higgins B, Gosal H. A correlation of time with meniscal tears in anterior cruciate ligament deficiency: stratifying the risk of surgical delay. *Knee Surg Sports Traumatol Arthrosc*. 2009;17(1):30-34.

58. Richmond JC, Lubowitz JH, Poehling GG. Prompt operative intervention reduces long-term osteoarthritis after knee anterior cruciate ligament tear. *Arthroscopy*. 2011;27(2):149-152.

59. Beynnon BD, Johnson RJ, Abate JA, Fleming BC, Nichols CE. Treatment of anterior cruciate ligament injuries, part I. *Am J Sports Med*. 2005;33(10):1579-1602.

60. Hetsroni I, Lyman S, Do H, Mann G, Marx RG. Symptomatic pulmonary embolism after outpatient arthroscopic procedures of the knee: the incidence and risk factors in 418,323 arthroscopies. *J Bone Joint Surg Br*. 2011;93(1):47-51.

61. Kartus J, Magnusson L, Stener S, Brandsson S, Eriksson BI, Karlsson J. Complications following arthroscopic anterior cruciate ligament reconstruction. A 2-5-year follow-up of 604 patients with special emphasis on anterior knee pain. *Knee Surg Sports Traumatol Arthrosc*. 1999;7(1):2-8.

62. Cullison TR, Muldoon MP, Gorman JD, Goff WB. The incidence of deep venous thrombosis in anterior cruciate ligament reconstruction. *Arthroscopy*. 1996;12(6):657-659.

63. Reinhardt KR, Hetsroni I, Marx RG. Graft selection for anterior cruciate ligament reconstruction: a level I systematic review comparing failure rates and functional outcomes. *Orthop Clin North Am*. 2010;41(2):249-262.

64. Bales CP, Guettler JH, Moorman CT,3rd. Anterior cruciate ligament injuries in children with open physes: evolving strategies of treatment. *Am J Sports Med*. 2004;32(8):1978-1985.

65. Halm EA, Lee C, Chassin MR. Is volume related to outcome in health care? A systematic review and methodologic critique of the literature. *Ann Intern Med*. 2002;137(6):511-520.

66. Katz JN, Losina E, Barrett J, et al. Association between hospital and surgeon procedure volume and outcomes of total hip replacement in the United States medicare population. *J Bone Joint Surg Am*. 2001;83-A(11):1622-1629.

67. Heck DA, Robinson RL, Partridge CM, Lubitz RM, Freund DA. Patient outcomes after knee replacement. *Clin Orthop Relat Res*. 1998;(356):93-110.

68. Norton EC, Garfinkel SA, McQuay LJ, et al. The effect of hospital volume on the in-hospital complication rate in knee replacement patients. *Health Serv Res.* 1998;33(5 Pt 1):1191-1210.

69. Taylor HD, Dennis DA, Crane HS. Relationship between mortality rates and hospital patient volume for Medicare patients undergoing major orthopaedic surgery of the hip, knee, spine, and femur. *J Arthroplasty.* 1997;12(3):235-242.

70. Birkmeyer JD, Stukel TA, Siewers AE, Goodney PP, Wennberg DE, Lucas FL. Surgeon volume and operative mortality in the United States. *N Engl J Med.* 2003;349(22):2117-2127.

71. Hillner BE, Smith TJ, Desch CE. Hospital and physician volume or specialization and outcomes in cancer treatment: importance in quality of cancer care. *J Clin Oncol.* 2000;18(11):2327-2340.

72. Jain N, Pietrobon R, Hocker S, Guller U, Shankar A, Higgins LD. The relationship between surgeon and hospital volume and outcomes for shoulder arthroplasty. *J Bone Joint Surg Am.* 2004;86-A(3):496-505.

73. Andersson C, Odensten M, Good L, Gillquist J. Surgical or non-surgical treatment of acute rupture of the anterior cruciate ligament. A randomized study with long-term follow-up. *J Bone Joint Surg Am.* 1989;71(7):965-974.

74. Borchers JR, Pedroza A, Kaeding C. Activity level and graft type as risk factors for anterior cruciate ligament graft failure: a case-control study. *Am J Sports Med.* 2009;37(12):2362-2367.

75. Fu FH. Double-bundle ACL reconstruction. *Orthopedics.* 2011; 34(4):281-283.

76. Yasuda K, van Eck CF, Hoshino Y, Fu FH, Tashman S. Anatomic single- and double-bundle anterior cruciate ligament reconstruction, part 1: basic science. *Am J Sports Med.* 2011;39(8):1789-1799.

77. Pombo MW, Shen W, Fu FH. Anatomic double-bundle anterior cruciate ligament reconstruction: where are we today? *Arthroscopy.* 2008;24(10):1168-1177.

78. Fu FH, Shen W, Starman JS, Okeke N, Irrgang JJ. Primary anatomic double-bundle anterior cruciate ligament reconstruction: a preliminary 2-year prospective study. *Am J Sports Med.* 2008;36(7):1263-1274.

79. Meredick RB, Vance KJ, Appleby D, Lubowitz JH. Outcome of single-bundle versus double-bundle reconstruction of the anterior cruciate ligament: a meta-analysis. *Am J Sports Med.* 2008;36(7):1414-1421.

80. Kohen RB, Sekiya JK. Single-bundle versus double-bundle posterior cruciate ligament reconstruction. *Arthroscopy.* 2009; 25(12):1470-1477.

81. Gobbi A, Mahajan V, Karnatzikos G, Nakamura N. Single- versus double-bundle ACL reconstruction: is there any difference in stability and function at 3-year followup? *Clin Orthop Relat Res.* 2012;470(3):824-834.

82. Suomalainen P, Moisala AS, Paakkala A, Kannus P, Jarvela T. Double-Bundle Versus Single-Bundle Anterior Cruciate Ligament Reconstruction: Randomized Clinical and Magnetic Resonance Imaging Study With 2-Year Follow-up. *Am J Sports Med.* 2011;39(8):1615-1622.

83. Shelbourne KD, Urch SE. Primary anterior cruciate ligament reconstruction using the contralateral autogenous patellar tendon. *Am J Sports Med.* 2000;28(5):651-658.

84. Shelbourne KD, Vanadurongwan B, Gray T. Primary anterior cruciate ligament reconstruction using contralateral patellar tendon autograft. *Clin Sports Med.* 2007;26(4):549-565.

85. Kocher MS, Garg S, Micheli LJ. Physeal sparing reconstruction of the anterior cruciate ligament in skeletally immature prepubescent children and adolescents. *J Bone Joint Surg Am.* 2005;87(11):2371-2379.

86. Vavken P, Murray MM. Treating anterior cruciate ligament tears in skeletally immature patients. *Arthroscopy.* 2011;27(5):704-716.

87. Guzzanti V, Falciglia F, Stanitski CL. Physeal-sparing intraarticular anterior cruciate ligament reconstruction in preadolescents. *Am J Sports Med.* 2003;31(6):949-953.

88. Schub D, Saluan P. Anterior cruciate ligament injuries in the young athlete: evaluation and treatment. *Sports Med Arthrosc.* 2011;19(1):34-43.

89. Kocher MS, Garg S, Micheli LJ. Physeal sparing reconstruction of the anterior cruciate ligament in skeletally immature pre-pubescent children and adolescents. Surgical technique. *J Bone Joint Surg Am.* 2006;88 Suppl 1 Pt 2:283-293.

90. Lo IK, Kirkley A, Fowler PJ, Miniaci A. The outcome of operatively treated anterior cruciate ligament disruptions in the skeletally immature child. *Arthroscopy.* 1997;13(5):627-634.

91. Lyman S, Hetsroni I, Do H, Marx RG. Meniscectomy After Meniscal Repair. Abstract presented at ISAKOS conference, May 19, 2011.

92. McCarty EC, Marx RG, DeHaven KE. Meniscus repair: considerations in treatment and update of clinical results. *Clin Orthop Relat Res.* 2002;(402):122-134.

93. Fanelli GC, Stannard JP, Stuart MJ, et al. Management of complex knee ligament injuries. *Instr Course Lect.* 2011;60:523-535.

94. Maak TG, Marx RG, Wickiewicz TL. Management of chronic tibial subluxation in the multiple-ligament injured knee. *Sports Med Arthrosc.* 2011;19(2):147-152.

95. Levy BA, Dajani KA, Whelan DB, et al. Decision making in the multiligament-injured knee: an evidence-based systematic review. *Arthroscopy.* 2009;25(4):430-438.

96. Levy BA, Fanelli GC, Whelan DB, et al. Controversies in the treatment of knee dislocations and multiligament reconstruction. *J Am Acad Orthop Surg.* 2009;17(4):197-206.

97. Marx RG, Hetsroni I. Surgical technique: medial collateral ligament reconstruction using achilles allograft for combined knee ligament injury. *Clin Orthop Relat Res.* 2012;470(3):798-805.

98. Marx RG. Functional bracing was no better than nonbracing after anterior cruciate ligament repair. *J Bone Joint Surg Am.* 2005;87(8):1890.

99. Wright RW, Preston E, Fleming BC, et al. A systematic review of anterior cruciate ligament reconstruction rehabilitation: part I: continuous passive motion, early weight bearing, postoperative bracing, and home-based rehabilitation. *J Knee Surg.* 2008;21(3):217-224.

100. Shelbourne KD, Gray T. Anterior cruciate ligament reconstruction with autogenous patellar tendon graft followed by accelerated rehabilitation. A two- to nine-year followup. *Am J Sports Med.* 1997;25(6):786-795.

101. Shelbourne KD, Nitz P. Accelerated rehabilitation after anterior cruciate ligament reconstruction. *Am J Sports Med.* 1990;18(3):292-299.

102. Myklebust G, Maehlum S, Engebretsen L, Strand T, Solheim E. Registration of cruciate ligament injuries in Norwegian top level team handball. A prospective study covering two seasons. *Scand J Med Sci Sports.* 1997;7(5):289-292.

103. Myklebust G, Maehlum S, Holm I, Bahr R. A prospective cohort study of anterior cruciate ligament injuries in elite Norwegian team handball. *Scand J Med Sci Sports.* 1998;8(3):149-153.

104. Cerulli G, Benoit DL, Caraffa A, Ponteggia F. Proprioceptive training and prevention of anterior cruciate ligament injuries in soccer. *J Orthop Sports Phys Ther.* 2001;31(11):655-60; discussion 661.

105. Koga H, Nakamae A, Shima Y, et al. Mechanisms for noncontact anterior cruciate ligament injuries: knee joint kinematics in 10 injury situations from female team handball and basketball. *Am J Sports Med.* 2010;38(11):2218-2225.

106. Arnason A, Andersen TE, Holme I, Engebretsen L, Bahr R. Prevention of hamstring strains in elite soccer: an intervention study. *Scand J Med Sci Sports.* 2008;18(1):40-48.

107. Cicuttini FM, Forbes A, Yuanyuan W, Rush G, Stuckey SL. Rate of knee cartilage loss after partial meniscectomy. *J Rheumatol.* 2002;29(9):1954-1956.

108. Roos EM. Joint injury causes knee osteoarthritis in young adults. *Curr Opin Rheumatol.* 2005;17(2):195-200.

109. Rotterud JH, Sivertsen EA, Forssblad M, Engebretsen L, Aroen A. Effect of gender and sports on the risk of full-thickness articular cartilage lesions in anterior cruciate ligament-injured knees: a nationwide cohort study from Sweden and Norway of 15 783 patients. *Am J Sports Med.* 2011;39(7):1387-1394.

110. Paterno MV, Schmitt LC, Ford KR, et al. Biomechanical measures during landing and postural stability predict second anterior cruciate ligament injury after anterior cruciate ligament reconstruction and return to sport. *Am J Sports Med.* 2010;38(10):1968-1978.

111. MARS Group, Wright RW, Huston LJ, et al. Descriptive epidemiology of the Multicenter ACL Revision Study (MARS) cohort. *Am J Sports Med.* 2010;38(10):1979-1986.

112. Magnussen RA, Granan LP, Dunn WR, et al. Cross-cultural comparison of patients undergoing ACL reconstruction in the United States and Norway. *Knee Surg Sports Traumatol Arthrosc.* 2010;18(1):98-105.

113. DeHaven KE, Lintner DM. Athletic injuries: comparison by age, sport, and gender. *Am J Sports Med.* 1986;14(3):218-224.

114. Mohtadi NG, Webster-Bogaerts, Fowler PJ. Limitation of motion following anterior cruciate ligament reconstruction. A case-control study. *Am J Sports Med.* 1991;19(6):620-624.

INDEX